ESSAYS FROM AN UNFINISHED PHYSICIAN

lessons from PEOPLE, PATIENTS, and LIFE

E. GREY DIMOND, M.D.

Authors Choice Press
San Jose New York Lincoln Shanghai

Essays From An Unfinished Physician
Lessons From People, Patients, and Life

All Rights Reserved © 1994, 2000 by Diastole-Hospital Hill, Inc.

No part of this book may be reproduced or transmitted in any form or by any means, graphic, electronic, or mechanical, including photocopying, recording, taping, or by any information storage or retrieval system, without the permission in writing from the publisher.

Authors Choice Press
an imprint of iUniverse.com, Inc.

For information address:
iUniverse.com, Inc.
5220 S 16th, Ste. 200
Lincoln, NE 68512
www.iuniverse.com

Originally published by Diastole

ISBN: 0-595-14788-7

Printed in the United States of America

DEDICATION

This volume is dedicated to the three deans who escorted the School from its founding to the present: Founding Dean Richardson K. Noback, Dean Harry S. Jonas, Dean James J. Mongan.

AND TO THE GRADUATES

ACKNOWLEDGMENTS

The working draft of this manuscript was read by Dr. James J. Mongan, Dr. Ben J. Wilson, E. Virginia Calkins, Jill Alexander, and James L. Soward. Their criticisms and suggestions are appreciated.

ESSAYS FROM AN UNFINISHED PHYSICIAN

SCOPE

I. THE ROLE OF A PHYSICIAN
twelve essays

II. HEALTH CARE REFORM
seven essays

III. ON MEDICAL EDUCATION
seven essays

IV. LESSONS FROM LIFE'S EXPERIENCES
fourteen essays

V. HOBBIES, INTERESTS, DOGS, TURTLES, WOODCARVING, AND THE RUBAIYAT
six essays

VI. INTERESTS ABROAD
nine essays

VII. TYING IT ALL TOGETHER
eight essays

ESSAYS FROM AN UNFINISHED PHYSICIAN

TABLE OF CONTENTS

I. THE ROLE OF A PHYSICIAN

ETHICS
1. Above and Beyond
   ... additional ethical burdens of physicians
2. On Behalf of Elitism
   ... crisis in medicine, the high ground

LEARNING
3. Life's Theater
   ... learning from patients
4. I'm Losing My Whacko
   ... the human variable, strange cases

DOCTOR'S ROLE
5. The Pursuit of Happiness
   ... the unremitting truth

STRESS
6. Happily Stressed
   ... the value of stress

OUTSIDE INTERESTS
7. Pencils
   ... save time for yourself

VACATION
8. Time for Smelling the Flowers
   ... back away from the duty

AGE
9. Wax Museum
   ... stuffed, waxed, ready

10. Age and Administration
    ... doing the right thing at the right time
11. Osler and Old Age
    ... good advice doesn't grow old
12. The Unchanging Role
    ... the eternal role of the physician

II. HEALTH REFORM

COST ISSUE
13. Our Choice: Illth or Health
    ... medical costs will never be contained
14. No Price Tag
    ... why should they be contained?
POLITICS
15. Compromised Health Care
    ... special interests in health reform
CHANGES
16. Living, Loving, and Dying
    ... be careful with change and cost containment
17. Doc-in-the-Box
    ... humor helps the pain
THE DOCTOR'S ROLE
18. Physicians and Politics
    ... get involved
19. The High Road
    ... the high road, the physician's road

III. MEDICAL EDUCATION

PRE-MED
20. On Becoming Civilized
    ... living is a liberal education

SELECTION
21. Mirror, Mirror on the Wall
    ... no magic rule for choosing
TEACHING
22. Peer Status
    ... lessons not forgot
CURRICULUM
23. Curriculum Packing
    ... don't overload the curriculum
LESSONS FROM TEACHING
24. The Touch of Greatness
    ... an exposure to greatness
25. Hunkerin' Down
    ... learning while teaching
GRADUATION ADVICE
26. Ten Minutes -- Five Words
    ... advice on commencing your life

IV. LESSONS FROM LIFE

YOUTH
27. Lessons from Shortstop
    ... all men are not created equal
28. Peaches Ellis
    ... experience and leadership
29. Moral: Beware of Greed
    ... take some lessons and learn the game
30. Tabasco Sauce and Cold Beer
    ... try almost everything -- carefully
YOUNG ADULT
31. On Building Character
    ... physical labor is physical labor
32. Knowing When to Cut
    ... on taking right angle turns

HOSPITAL HILL
33. Poll Taking on Hospital Hill
   ... can good be found in pollution?
34. Gardening in the City
   ... an inner city island

LIFE'S SCARS, LIFE'S LESSONS
35. The Battlefield
   ... lessons from the body's scars
36. This is Liberation?
   ... women and life's juggling act
37. Tourist Class
   ... it is difficult to be noble

FRIENDSHIPS
38. Friendship
   ... my Japanese physician
39. Father John
   ... one must gather these like a bouquet
40. Me and My Shadow
   ... when young, the long view is hazy

V. HOBBIES AND INTERESTS

PETS
41. MaMa is a He
   ... save room for a dog
42. Chance? Fate?
   ... and more room
43. Mississippi Yellow Ear Retires
   ... think carefully before acquiring a turtle

CARVING
44. Shaping Wood
   ... on using the hands
45. Roots, Kansas, Lea Grey
   ... the south wind

COLLECTING
46. Rubaiyatiana
    ... the reward of collecting

VI. INTERESTS ABROAD

TIBET
47. Xigatse Stress Test
    ... religion, the hard way
48. The Joy of the Journey
    ... a graduation gift for all

MOSCOW
49. Forty-three Hours in Moscow
    ... not even time for jet lag

CHINA
50. Basic Hopes and Fears
    ... one-fourth of mankind
51. Why?
    ... the oldest, largest civilization
52. What is the Margin of Truth?
    ... separating fact from propaganda
53. More Than Herbs and Acupuncture
    ... good enough for grandmother
54. The Return of China
    ... China's return and the 21st century
55. Simmons Fred Slept Here
    ... two great nations, two ways of speaking

VII. TYING IT TOGETHER

56. Eternal Verities
    ... time and place change, but the truth endures
57. All Hung Out: Shore-to-Shore
    ... stay steady, the cycle will turn

58. Obits to Match Our Mountains
    ... the merit of proper endings
59. Verbal Speed and Obsolescence
    ... on gaps and generations
60. On Hard Work and Being "Educated"
    ... beware of established literature
61. Care and Maintenance of the Body
    ... there are no trade-ins
62. Some Secrets
    ... don't feel you must fit the pattern
63. Age 70
    ... living is an education

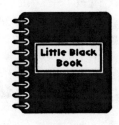

INTRODUCTION

You are holding a collection of personal opinions about living, loving, dying, and way stations inbetween. Opinions about duty, purpose, commitment, and the world physicians live in are expressed in an archaic form of communication: the brief essay. The reader may be sure that these essays are biased, opinionated, even a bit autocratic. The author has been a physician for 50 years, an experience guaranteed to mean that the essays are about patients and medical care, managed or otherwise. I do not write as pro-national health legislation or against it. I believe in personal, devoted duty and define it as the privilege of the bedside. However, other things make up a physician's life, too. Part of the joy of the journey included good living time with dogs, baseball, golf, football, travel, family, friends, books, whackos, acupuncture -- and other things.

In these 50 years of doctoring, I wandered from the bedside frequently and founded a new medical school, helped create the largest education institution in the world for heart doctors, served a year and half apprenticeship in the political process in Washington, led U.S. State Department-sponsored teaching groups of physicians to 20 countries, was in and out of Asia forty times, including being in the first group of physicians in China after 22 years of the Bamboo Curtain, taught clinical medicine to practicing physicians at a twice a year, ten day retreat for 30 years, produced a monthly one hour audiotape for physicians for 18 consecutive years, and wrote a once a month essay for medical students, their parents, and physicians for 25 years.

None of that proves that the opinions expressed are right. Perhaps they do verify that the writer has survived exposure to very critical audiences.

The medical profession has been placed on the defensive in recent years. All about us the media keep nipping. I have been deep in every role of modern medicine from direct practice, to research, to teaching the student, the graduate student, the practitioner. Add government medicine, grant-getting medicine, international medicine, medical school and hospital administration. All of this at least qualifies me for an opinion -- and at the same time leaves me vulnerable to the criticism of bias.

Bias? of course, I am biased. This book is Medicine as I have seen it, as my students have heard it, as I taught men and women in practice. The truth is that the public is very well-served by a dedicated core of physicians. That is my primary message.

The United States is politicking its way into some version of national health care. I have enjoyed every aspect of a physician's life and believe there are very basic truths about ethics, morality, kindness, and caring that must be protected. These essays are tied together by that theme.

As you read, you will note the audience is often medical. Enjoy that approach. Looking at the medical profession from the inside can be beneficial.

My house is on a hill, Hospital Hill. The name of my home is *Diastole*. Down the hill from *Diastole* are our medical school and hospitals.

Diastole takes its name from that period in the heart's cycle when the heart is at rest. I considered the long years of practice and teaching as Systole, the period in which the heart works. My years of Systole have brought me to *Diastole*.

E. Grey Dimond, M. D.
Diastole
Hospital Hill
Kansas City, Missouri   64108

I. THE ROLE OF A PHYSICIAN

1. Above and Beyond

There is much written and said about ethics and conduct. This is a choice area for criticism of our profession. It is easy to become irritated at those all about us, not physicians, who so enthusiastically define these areas. However, becoming irritated serves no value, and the truth is that the physician is an agent of society, and does work in an area of living and dying. Standards, rules, conduct, ethics are defined for others: real estate brokers, lawyers, politicians -- yes, they do have standards. Society does understand that only one profession is a matter of life and death.

I am so fond of our profession and have such deep respect for it that I do have difficulty accepting that an "outsider," someone not a physician, can, even should, tell me what is right and what is wrong. After an initial moment of flare, I settle back and know that we, the profession, do not make the rules nor set the standards for what is acceptable.

Two areas quickly make clear what I mean. Abortion and euthanasia. Society, the people, not the profession, have the duty, the right, to define their expectation. The fact that "they" define it does not automatically mean the physician must accept the duty to "do" it. A law made by legislators requiring a physician to administer the lethal medicaments for execution does not meet my own standard of ethics. Thus, society may define -- but the physician reserves the moral decision.

My image, my expectation of our profession, is just that: We live under rules set by society, but we live by higher rules than society defines. Does this mean that physicians are beyond the law? A critic could say that this is self-serving, an aggrandizement of our profession. Perhaps it is. However, the public would be poorly served if all we did was live by the rules. It is the gray areas where the rules are not defined, that the internal code of honor, of conduct, of the individual physician must be above the standards expected by society.

An English physician, Theodore Fox, for 40 years the conscience of the medical journal *The Lancet*, defined in his Harveian Oration in 1965 two rules that have guided me. He claimed that the primary task of a physician is to help people rather than to advance science. This is a truth not always remembered by those who create medical curriculum or who make judgments on the quality of a medical school.

His second belief was that nations do allow physicians to have a more advanced code than their own society's code. For the majority, there is a national quality of patriotism, or national expectation of ultimate conduct. But " ... nations do indicate, do allow, that medicine has a more advanced code than their national own ... the doctor is right to put his duty to the human race before his duty to any of its components' groups. However uncertain and tentative, the physician is a prototype of a supranational man."

"A more advanced code than their national own." That is a rule for physicians worth living by.

2. On Behalf of Elitism

Our profession, Medicine, is in a crisis time: Those in medical school are hearing the steady lament that there are too many physicians. Those in residency hear there are too many specialists in the very field they are entering. The physician in practice is living through an experience unlike any of the past. The civic spirit that created and sustained the community hospital is replaced by an anonymous, unseen, stock-held corporation.

The very hospitals are entering the practice of medicine, becoming the employer of the physician. The opportunity to practice independent, "solo" private practice is ending. Compensation for one's professional services is determined by others, not the physician. His income decreases, the number of patients decreases, the accessibility of the hospital decreases. The rewards are decreased, the punishment increased -- a malpractice suit is a hovering specter.

Where does the physician turn to find a rallying point? Does he become a salaried 40-hour-a-week corporate employee? Does he rally by using the tactic of unionizing? Do his organizations, the AMA and his own specialty college, become the defenders, or are they made impotent by federal trade rulings? Is it all a futile battle with the best response being the quietest one?

Should the physician accept these changes and go on taking care of those who come for care, letting the means of compensation, of authority change -- but hold fast, at least trying, to the basic commitment: serve the patient?

I do not offer any answers except that which I have written and spoken of repeatedly: Take to the high ground. In this all-people-are-equal, populous-oriented society, I raise a flag, a rallying cry, for the cause of Elitism.

Before falling under the arrows, I cry out, "Yes! Equality for all! Equal at birth and all become unequal as fast as their natural abilities can bring it about!" I must plead guilty to a firm belief that life is a competitive endeavor and the race belongs to the swift -- of intellect, swift of ambition and, in medicine, swift in one's concern for fellow man.

Thomas Jefferson, a substantial elitist, said, "There is a natural aristocracy among men. The grounds of this are virtue and talent." That expresses my sentiment -- let virtue be expressed as caring, as compassion, and talent as intellect strengthened by ambition.

Those who attack and criticize the word elitism are faulting another overtone, a designation of position and rank because it was handed down by family. Of course, that is not my message.

I specify a natural aristocracy, natural as a set of personal qualities, of personal virtue and talent. Who faults that? I don't refer to a position due to family or money.

The times and circumstances affecting the practice of medicine are involved in high rates of change. There is an unshakable basis for that Jeffersonian elitist practicing with virtue and talent. There is a privilege which the marketing experts, the promoters, the profit-makers, the economists cannot gain, and that is the privilege of the bedside, the actual right to serve people. Let that be our concern, our dedication, our virtue.

There is the high ground. There we must rally, concentrating our purpose on service, jealous only of the patient's well-being. The privilege of the bedside is the high ground.

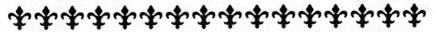

3. Life's Theater

In the beginning there is a medical student and the first major patient experience. All schools have this moment of initiation. Fresh, excited, apprehensive, worried more about embarrassment than about failure, the student begins the long initiation. The problems defined in book and lecture now become human beings. Life as physician has begun.

Medical school passes; the residency years bring more immersion in the arena of human problems. Finally the point of "going into practice" comes. The medical student has become a trained physician, but the freshness, the excitement, the apprehension remain.

The years of commitment continue; we call it the practice of medicine, but it could be called "living theater." All the material, the grist, the imagination used by novelists and playwrights are real life, daily life for the physician.

They come, one at a time. Sick, worried, frightened, vulnerable -- angry, hostile, conniving, cheating, faltering, confiding, lying, manipulating, scheming. They come, one at a time, in some way leaning on the shoulder of the physician. They lean, talk, tell, expose. They take away a part of the physician's basic faith in people.

The contact leaves both the patient and the physician changed. Someplace in the encounter the physician does something for the patient, for that is the nature of the transaction. Some knowledge, solace, advice, encouragement passes. One patient at a time is a very personal business.

The physician is not left unchanged. A lifetime

of serving the sick eventually alters the physician, more than we usually write about or speak. From the physician's very close-up, personal view of the individual human flaws, weaknesses, subterfuges, it is difficult to not arrive near the end as a cynic, a cynic about the human race. How did the poet word this? " ... I sit in my seat beside the road and hurl the cynics ban ... "

A now popular term, "burnout," does not exactly describe this change. It is an honest using up of the physician's milk, the milk of human kindness. The intimacy of medicine, personal care medicine, uses up the reservoir of one's love of mankind. One of my own teachers found this so true that he would sit in his darkened office, at the end of a full day of seeing patients, breathing in and out, finding solace in his pipe, and through clinched teeth would declare his final dictum: "People are no damn good."

There is another pathway that a lifetime of one-patient-at-a-time may open for the physician. Not cynicism, not technical aloofness -- but an education about the human condition, and from that comes a tolerance of the whole spectrum of peoplekind. One acquires a sense of joy about the untidy events of living, loving, and dying.

What other experience brings the observer into such a privileged view of his fellows? For some, such a journey creates a cynic. Some become a buffered technocrat who personally is unseen by the patient and does not experience the give and take of personal-care medicine.

Out of this lifetime crucible can emerge a wise person, seeing, experiencing life from a high, favored plateau. From feeling the pathos, but also the bravery, the humanness of it all, can come the acceptance of the wonderful drama, the need to expect all the variations and accept that there are those who cannot be enjoyed, only pitied. Cynicism? No, nor defeat.

If one can keep an open mind, a willingness to accept the illogic and confusion of much of it, the matured physician enjoys the theater with tolerance, love, laughter, and finds strength and adequate purpose for it all.

The time one has is limited. Try to do a bit of good, avoid harm, beware of anger, for if circumstances were changed, you and the other person would probably be friends. Take it all seriously, but not too much so. The ability to laugh is as important as the ability to be generous. Times change but your role in the living theater is the privileged one.

4. I'm Losing My Whacko

All physicians see mystery cases, the patient whose problem eludes them. The case you could not explain -- wondering what that odd collection of signs, symptoms, and tests should have said.

I saw a young Kansas farmer who deliberately starved and exercised himself through push-ups, chin-ups, etc., until he was reduced to 80 pounds. When I saw him he was cadaverous, bones covered by skin, and, although from a prosperous Kansas farm rich with food, was a prototype of the awfulness of concentration camps. Wasted as he was, he could struggle through two dozen push-ups. I saw him because he had a slow heart beat, a not uncommon happening in cases of starvation. An interesting example of how the wrong doctor sees the wrong patient. Or perhaps it was best. For I developed a friendship of sorts with him, assuring him about his heart, and learned that his real problem was different from what I remotely expected. He was convinced that his penis was disappearing within him, and he had fasted and exercised in an effort to tighten up his body around the disappearing organ. He did not use the word penis but said in a whisper, "I'm losing my whacko."

This was not a problem that I had any knowledge about but after reassuring him about his slow heart beat, I was able to reason with him, and over a period of a year gained his confidence that his nether parts would remain with him. When I last saw him he weighed 160 pounds, whacko and all. I put his "before" and "after" photographs and electrocardiograms in a textbook on electrocardiography and knew I had not exactly understood what I had seen.

Time passed, 30 years in fact, and the experience remained stuck in memory as something not understood. Then *The Lancet* had a letter to the editor from the All-India Institutes of Medical Sciences and it said: "Sir: Koro is an acute anxiety reaction in which the patient fears that his or her genitalia are shrinking and may disappear into the abdomen ... " There! At last an answer for my young Kansas farmer: Koro. It of course helps me not at all simply to have a label, but it helps to know that such human experience has occurred often enough to have entered the literature. The letter from India was stimulated by an epidemic, yes epidemic, of Koro in northeast India. The physicians there had recognized it as a group hysteria. Of course there is just as much logic for an epidemic of Koro as there was for the epidemic of the original St. Vitus Dance, or the swooning of teenagers in the presence of an entertainment idol.

The Indian authors report that in a period of a few weeks, 60 cases occurred in villages comprising 600 households. The native healers had given it the name and claimed they had a cure. The cure was one that would get the attention of anyone with this problem of disappearing genitalia: "To hold the 'affected' part tightly, while cold water is poured over the head, and give the patient lime juice to drink." I don't believe my Kansas farmer would have appreciated this advice but having this reference may be therapeutic if I ever see a case of the disappearing whacko again.

5. The Pursuit of Happiness

The theme of the merchandising carried on by marketing experts charged with filling hospital beds is: "We care. Come to us for the personal attention your cold, technical specialist has deprived you of. We are holistically yours; all our thoughts are devoted to the complete you. Not only all parts of you, but holistically all parts of your wife, mother, aunt, children. We care."

I realize that a great deal of this talk is a part of the popular enthusiasm for what is called alternative healing, which includes organic foods, no additives, transcendental meditation, yoga, wushi, taichi, acupuncture, aloes, Zen, incense, sandals, massage, gurus, and reincarnation. I admit that I threw a lot into my definition of holisticism and I may be guilty of taking a blow at a few things that get involved by association.

The message I seek to develop is that one serves their body poorly if, because of a desire for holistic, warm, personal attention, one turns away from the immense range of scientific diagnosis, medical and surgical care.

There is no doubt it is high-tech, no doubt it is expensive -- the machines cost fortunes, and no one has a way of making them free. Next season's machines will be better and still not free.

For the moment, I set aside the question of the cost of care and speak only of the ability of modern technology to aid and prolong life. Physicians need to get off the defensive about the cold, high-technology, equipment-oriented nature of modern medicine. It is high-tech. It will get more so. It saves lives. The interventions, the invasions bring life-enhancing benefits.

Economists cry warnings that the cost of medical care now exceeds 14 percent of the national budget. That fact is cited with alarm. Why is it not just as reasonable to consider it a bargain? What should society do? Cancel these new, better -- much better -- tools? There is a cry that we must begin rationing who gets access to these expensive health measures. It is urgently stated that no nation can afford unlimited medical care, and self-appointed experts, grandstand ethicists, self-importantly declare society must make decisions about who is inside the care corral and who, by decision, is outside.

All of this leaves me cold. My thinking is so clear and the answers seem so logical that I can't but wonder why all the discussion.

For those who want an alternative form of care, no matter how illogical, let that be their choice. If what they want does not risk the rest of us, then have no concern. Let them buy what they want. If they insist that the wind in their hair while riding their motorcycles is their business, not society's, arrest them. Their exposed skulls are our business.

For those who must smoke, let them smoke. Raise the price of tobacco immensely, put the revenue in a trust fund -- they'll be back and need it. Of course, maintain a prohibition on advertising the poison and propagandize constantly about the lethalness of smoking. Does this interfere with freedom? No more than insisting that it is your right to drive always on the wrong side of the street.

For most of us, staying well and alive is just about the overriding value with which we deal. Very technical, very complicated modern medicine has the best promise of accomplishing that. Who can put a percent of GNP value on the cost of life, liberty, and the pursuit of happiness?

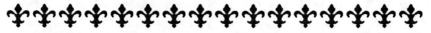

6. Happily Stressed

Living is stressful and stress is a useful condition. With this opening sentence, I know I am inviting bricks and stones.

The world is rich with messages that stress is destructive. Enthusiastic therapy is offered by anti-stress specialists. A serene, stress-free condition is extolled as the sublime state. Relax! Stretch! Fish! Golf! Massage. Vibrators. Rolfing. Biofeedback. Inhale. Transcend. Meditate. And vegetate.

The truth is that the world's progress depends upon well-stressed, highly enthusiastic, intelligent people not yet 40. Progress is the key word. Older people contribute, regulate, administer. However, the original bursts of new creative talent are brought forward from those who are on the rushing, all-out energetic side of life, those wonderful years between 20 and 40.

Osler said that the great deeds are done by those who have the sun on their brow, not on their back. A quite poetic way, relating life, career, and time.

The DNA discoverer, Nobel laureate James Watson, when younger, said that unique, original, creative research work was done before age 30. He managed his research institute by this rule, and talent rushed, bustled, and created -- then, shortly after 30, were on their way to more staid years at other institutions. He felt comfortable that he had already harvested their best years. Later he moved the cut-off to 40 years but now, as he reached his own retirement, he held to his conviction that 40 is the closing down of one's unique, energetic, creative time.

Now that I have made most of my senior colleagues wince, I hurry to remind that the full-blown after-40 years are the years of judgment, wisdom, leadership, steadiness. Osler and Watson speak of the fires of spring, those rare precious years in which time has no limit, energy pours forth, and experience has not yet taught barriers.

Now that I have savored, used, spent the whole allotted spectrum of years, I cast my vote on those wonderful days before 40. What rewards, what pleasure they can bring. What a waste one can make of them. How precious and unretrievable they are.

Stress can be awful; I well understand its limits and that each of us has a breaking point. However, when you are young, and you are fully prepared for your profession, and your talent is directed in an altruistic field such as medicine, and when the rewards are satisfying, then there is no destructive stress.

It is a useful, needed, stimulating condition and one which will bring forth the finest within you. Stress is painful for those who are overmatched. Stress for a young physician is an honorable provocateur, an internal ally, that will multiply your natural talents and the training which has prepared you. Enjoy stress! Worry, get restless when it is missing.

7. Pencils

I don't in the least believe the medical degree requires a pulling of shades around the larger world. Very bright minds are restless minds. Medical discipline does not constrain the range of one's enthusiasm. An aphorism of life is that those who get things done--are those who gets things done.

You discover that whether you do a little or do a lot, you will fill up a 24-hour day. No more, no less. The work you do will expand to fill your schedule. Whether very much done or very little, one gets up in the morning and goes to bed at night. What you do in between is called living.

I write about living outside the practice of medicine. Sir William Osler cautioned young medical graduates with the words, "Medicine is a jealous mistress." For his time and circumstance that was a quite racy comparison. He was warning those about to become physicians of how much energy and commitment are needed. He was equally saying that those we care for will have an unlimited demand upon our time.

Osler's remark is a reminder to a young doctor to be aware of how much she or he should give to this all-consuming profession. The demands are so great in the early years that encouragement to pace yourself seems unreal. When one is running all out to stay ahead of the tiger, remarks about the scenery make the runner angry -- or dead.

From being a student to being a prepared physician is a journey beyond anticipation. It is a hard journey, one fully occupying time and energy. Success and prosperity are rewards one can expect. They come. My caution is to hold back time, hold back some part of life for other growing.

To be an able, wise physician at mid-life requires a giving by oneself but it must not exhaust enthusiasm, nor willingness to serve. It is easy to be burned up, burned out, by the obligations carried by a physician. To give everything one has means there is nothing left. Life is a long trip; intellectual baggage acquired at the beginning will need replenishing, so will the physician. Willingness to continue for a lifetime the discipline of serving means one must find ways of refreshing and recharging.

A painful, grinding way to understand what it means to be a physician is to compare you, your career, to a pencil, and the ability of patients to consume you, to a pencil sharpener. The rate at which you are consumed depends almost entirely upon the pressure placed on the pencil as it is pushed into the whirling, grinding, consuming machine. Without caution, without easing up on the pressure, the pencil quickly disappears. Nothing but the shavings remain. Yet the sharpener, the patients' needs, remain ready, whirling, willing, to consume the next pressed pencil. Life for a physician is painfully similar. Learn the pressure that keeps the pencil sharpened, but learn when to pull back.

Learn to ease yourself with travel, with theater, with sports, art, collecting, your children, the one you love. Learn a thousand ways to expand yourself. Such things are sometimes called hobbies, but they are habits, therapeutic habits which sustain you and lessen the exhaustion, the all-encompassing requirements of being a good physician.

Pace your use of life, find a level of service that gives the best of yourself. Leave time for your own growth. At 24, 44 seems remote. But it is only tomorrow. Plan your journey so you arrive at each way-station strong, enthusiastic, able -- and wiser.

There is very little use for an eraser connected to a 1-inch pencil.

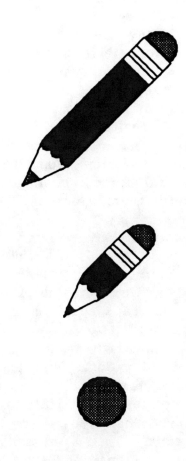

8. Time for Smelling the Flowers

I have just finished a bona-fide vacation. I use the expression "bona fide" to separate this two-week period from so many other semi-vacations which physicians snatch from their complex lives. Semi-vacations include those times spent combining attendance at a postgraduate course with breathing salt air, rushing off to a weekend medical retreat at a local hotel, playing medical tapes in the car, reading medical journals in a resort hotel room, or calling the office to check on Mrs. Smith. Some holiday.

Through skillful forgetting, I got away to two weeks of pure, unadulterated vacation. I forgot to put a stack of journals in my bag, I forgot my dictation machine, I forgot to tell my secretary where I would be. Here is my report on this forgetful adventure.

First, the stored-up catecholamines can't be turned off instantly. One burns them for the first 48 hours by telephone calls back home to complete unfinished details, and two nights of insomnia in which the mind continues to grind over the variety of projects left unfinished. Some wise person, I think it was Churchill, noted that a refreshing vacation comes not in doing "nothing," but in doing vigorously something entirely different from that which consumes you at work. This is the truth.

Put in medical terms, one doesn't turn off the catecholamines, those internal chemicals that keep our tension up to the stress of living, but must redirect them into pleasurable tasks. When one is on the demanding treadmill of daily duty, to do nothing sounds wonderful. To do nothing, I timidly suggest, is an invitation to desuetude, hebetude, lassitude, and general non-well-being: vegetabletude.

Hammering a golf ball, crunching a tennis ball,

pounding the Nikes for miles -- all are good examples of how the human organism finds health and happiness, not always from the game, perhaps, but in finding another non-usual way to burn the catecholamines.

When one is young (or younger) and consumed by the fatigue of getting a career started, how to use a vacation seems a foolish question. Just getting two days off is a laudable goal. Later (and later comes sooner than one expects) come the long, long years of career, family, duty as a physician and parent -- the prime years of the life for which one invests so much in preparation.

How to use those years with an effective plan for work, and time for other things? Call it play, break, time-off, vacation, sabbatical or whatever: there is a need for a waxing and waning, a period of all-out duty, and equally committed, a period of all-out doing something else.

Not only did Churchill give such advice, an equally Anglo-Saxon sage, Mother Goose, said, "All work and no play makes Jack a dull boy."

I won't try to debate or promote the advantages of backpacking in the High Sierras, wet-suit snorkeling, or chiseling something out of a chunk of wood, for all these activities have served me well. My message is to remind all, and especially those coming along behind us, that living is action, being is doing, and that a rhythm of life requires change, a charging and recharging. One must be very careful of trying to do nothing.

9. Wax Museum

Here in Kansas City, I offer myself as a museum piece for any collector seeking an unsullied sample of the pre-now era.

The enthusiasm for a new set of social rules has passed me by. I have avoided the "with-it, let-it-hang-out, do-my-own-thing, duyano, touchy-feely" years. No books on porno, hard-core or soft, have passed before my eyes. No go-go dancing, topless or bottomless splendor, no tri-sexual marvels, no Woodstockian festivals, hard rock or metal -- none of these mind-expanding glories have I seen.

All of this unbelievable mess, currently being inhaled and extolled, of violence, mayhem, bloodiness, strange and variant rampages of sex and drugs, screeching music with clandestine lyrics, determined attempts to justify versions of conduct by calling up on the reeling Bill of Rights -- all of this I have avoided.

No Oprah, even Donahue, have I seen.

My guess (hope?) is that the cycle will go full around, the pendulum will swing, the scales will balance -- and this present exercise in bad taste will pass. A period of honorable behavior, of prudent conduct, of personal reserve, of family will return.

Why this noble offering of myself? I think I am but one of a host of similar prudes, but the others are too busy getting duty done. My point is that the vast majority of physicians lead sane, conservative, private dedicated lives. The media nip at our outside flanks and make the profession seem far less than it is. One can not go through the long years of medical school, then residency and years of practice and be anything but calm, conservative, and cautious.

Medical science and calm judgment serve a critical role as our society works its way through this unhappy mix of violent behavior.

A challenge to this advocacy is to ask if such a conservator of attitudes can be a confidant to his contemporaries living out a new set of social rules. Almost without rules. Is some modern living so far afield that there is no fit?

Social rules may have gone to hell but there is a core involving kindness, honesty, love, faith, truth, respect, loyalty, and dependability. These values do not age, change, are become out-dated. It is within these unchanging tenets that the physician functions.

A physician lives within these fundamentals, dispensing scientific knowledge, tempered by awareness of the pressures and risks of the society in which we live -- but giving not an inch in what are the fundamental values. Minister, priest, religion offer this but only part of it. The added dimension is the application of science. No other profession has this charge, from no other source can the patient get such skills. Medicine and religion are not competitive. Faith and healing, healing and faith. Both are holding the fort.

10. Age and Administration

Life's moments of ceremony come automatically: birth and baptism, high-school graduation, college commencement, marriage vows, the children. At this point, things settle down to one day after another, just living and doing. Then, much sooner than seems appropriate, one is 65 years old, and by a logic that is a part of the tradition of the land, one is a "senior citizen," in the "golden years," authorized for Medicare and life in Sun City.

From the beginning of my professional career, this date has been on my agenda. True, I have not had any hidden desire to hasten this crossing of the bar, but quietly I have waited for this moment of gaining the other side of the river. Why? For what purpose this preoccupation with a moment of ceremony, a moment announcing legal old age?

Because I have wanted to be on both sides, before 65 and after, and see if I was still a believer in what I said at 35, 45, and 55, namely that academic administration and management should not be in the hands of those past 65.

Now, across that age myself, do I still believe what could have been evidence of youthful prejudice when I was younger? Yes! The running of organizations should be turned over to those in prime career. Administration of an academic setting is best done by those still fluid with ambition, eager to cause change. The caution of age balances poorly with the youthful vigor of the growing careers of students and faculty.

Physicians, a very special breed, have another very special problem: professional obsolescence. Medical knowledge and equipment are changing at a stupendous rate.

A generation ago, a senior physician earned a position of respect because he had acquired vast exposure to humankind's problems from experience and usually had acquired an equally significant degree of wisdom.

Now, medical things change so fast that one becomes 65 with a treasure-house of experience and wisdom, but with a bag of professional tricks and knowledge painfully dated.

It is this fact, plus the change in methods of practicing medicine, called the "commercialization and competition" style of medicine, that is adding a new urgency to age 65 for the physicians.

For the first time, the logic of continuing to practice and reaping the benefit of being the senior consulting opinion is counterbalanced by the likelihood of a lack of comfort with things new, and a competitive "advertising" style of practice that is not at all attractive. Retirement, even early retirement, has quite definitely become an attractive prospect for the practicing physician.

I began this essay with a simple purpose: to validate that when I was 35, I thought the administration and management of an academic institution should be in the hands of those in prime years, and now, 30 years later, standing on the far edge of the bridge, that still seems right and logical to me.

Being 65 does not require Sun City, but the reins of power should be passed to those coming behind.

11. William Osler and Age 60

In these essays I know I have failed one of the important tests of erudition. I have not quoted sufficiently Sir William Osler. A medical writer who does not attach himself to Osler is of suspect origin.

Today I join the team. I quote Osler.

Osler, in a farewell talk, commented on the merit of retirement for doctors past age 60. He even slipped in the possibility of elimination. His words were:

"My ... fixed idea is the uselessness of men above 60 years of age, and the incalculable benefit it would be in commercial, political, and in professional life, if, as a matter of course, men stopped work at this age. The teacher's life should have three periods: study until 25, investigation until 40, profession until 60, at which age I would have him retired on a double allowance. Whether Anthony Trollope's suggestion of ... chloroform should be carried out or not, I have become a little dubious, as my time is getting so short."

Osler's remarks were made at the farewell banquet in Baltimore as he was feted before leaving Hopkins, to become regius professor at Oxford. Perhaps his purpose was to soften his leaving by suggesting that Hopkins had already had his best years. However, the newspapers gave his comment lasting impact. The next day the headline read, "OSLER RECOMMENDS CHLOROFORM AT SIXTY."

The sentiment of Osler's words, *sans* chloroform, comes to me often as I listen to my colleagues who are in the latter years of their medical careers.

Almost daily, old friends tell me of the unpleasantness of practice as it has become burdened with litigation and hostile media; with unending paperwork, bureaucratic interference and second guessing; with patients sold and bought as corporate pawns; and with shrill, embarrassing marketing.

The demand that one practice with business efficiency, the message that old, trusted hospitals are being absorbed into unfathomable corporate structures, that thousands of patients are "bought" by one organization, "sold" by another, makes the care and tending of one's personal patients no longer attractive. Osler's words urging early retirement sound reasonable to my longtime friends. Their advice is bitter as they approach the ends of their careers. There is a steady message: "Don't study medicine. Don't choose a medical career. This is no longer an attractive way to spend your life."

I hear this and I know why they feel this way. For them, it is not the way they began their careers and it is no longer the joy that it once was. One cannot let it rest there. Is this still not the best way to use one's life? Will it not continue to be the closest one can come to being truly useful? Is there any other way one can rise each day, go to bed each night, and know that your efforts were only for the good of your fellowkind? Can there be any role that so completely combines knowledge, technical and scientific skill with compassion -- and for the purpose of bringing betterment to the individual served?

I hear my friends. I share their sorrow, even shock at what we are passing through. However, it is still the best way to use one's life. To quote Osler again, and balance the negation of his farewell remarks: "Medicine is the Queen of the Professions." With its present-day burdens, with its harassments and even embarrassments, it is still, and will be, the finest way to use one's time on stage.

⚜⚜⚜⚜⚜⚜⚜⚜⚜⚜⚜⚜⚜

12. The Unchanging Role

One's own problems determine the size of the world. Enthusiasm for wealth, power, fame motivates one on Monday. On Tuesday, a hard mass in the neck is found; the goals of Monday are gone, replaced by the single, personal dread. One's own problems determine the size of the world.

That place in the brain where is stored the thing called "me" is rich with ego, ambition, material wants, passion. Success is measured by satisfying these drives. One lump in the neck reduces those wants to trivia.

We Americans live by a document in which is the claim that we deserve life, liberty, and the pursuit of happiness. The happiness we pursue, the liberty we seek, contract to disappearance when that primary value, LIFE, is threatened.

A wise physician accepts an inadequacy to judge these limits. It is enough to understand that, for most of us, life is our final possession. When the world has been made very small by the mass in the neck, by the deep pain in the chest, by the sudden gush of blood, it is there, in the dark world of fear, that the unchanging role of the physician begins.

But there are unpredicted, unpremeditated experiences when the internal "me" rises above, goes beyond, and sacrifices self. Heroism, a flashing moment when one places service to others above personal survival, excites us, frightens us. Nations write their history books about such sacrifice. Wars are not the only stimulus. Everyday, someone does a heroic act, unknown, unarranged, unanticipated, and has an inch in the paper, seconds on television, and we all wonder inside if our "me" would have let us do a similar act, an act, which declares there are values larger than one's own life.

Physicians have no special skill or role in this almost spiritual act. We are, as all others, laymen in the understanding of self-sacrifice. With all others, we pause and, deep inside, say, "Would I?" We are but laymen, yet because we deal with life and maintaining it is our purpose, perhaps we think more often about its mystery.

II. ON HEALTH REFORM

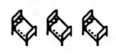

13. Our Choice: Illth or Health

From all sides we hear about the crisis and the cost of health care. My own objectivity is flawed. I am a physician with a full life of practice, teaching, research and administration -- all in the field of medicine.

From graduation in 1944 to the present gives me 50 years of duty. I observe the present discussion, the cries over cost, and think of the wonders I've seen.

Then, in the early '40s, we were taught to put the coronary occlusion patient in bed for six weeks; he could not feed himself, nor even shave. We learned how to put needles in the legs to get off the fluid of dropsy. We had absolutely no medication for hypertension. Now all of these calamities have direct life-saving solutions.

Cold, technical medicine? Balderdash. Technical scientific medicine is what made the change happen. I speak with knowledge in my own field, but every field of medicine has seen the same range of technical, scientific, interventional, pharmacological, expensive progress.

The old country doctor was no kinder; he simply had nothing else to offer but kindness.

The physician in the 1940s (me) gave the coronary patient morphine, darkened the room, put up a no visitors sign, and devoted time to consoling the family. Is that the kind of nostalgic care so often cited as missing? The cardiac catheter room, the operating room, and the recovery room are sterile, frightening. They are technical, they are mechanical, and they are expensive. But they are life.

Various efforts to hang guilt on physicians as the cause of medical care expense can be answered by some rather simple analysis. Neutralize the physicians' part of a nation's medical bill. Let us assume that all physicians were assigned a fixed annual stipend and no cost-of-living increase.

Would the cost of health care be contained? No. The progress in scientific advances would drive the marketplace, even with the elimination of the doctor variable. Not esoteric, unwarranted progress, but the same kind of progress that goes on now and yesterday.

Instead of cane-and-chair existence, we now have joint replacements.

Instead of near blindness, we have implanted lenses for cataracts; instead of death or incapacity, we have clot resolution, coronary angioplasty, bypass surgery.

For all of these, it was cheaper to leave the patient alone. A $9 cane, a wheelchair, lessons in Braille, or for the coronary patient, death -- those were solutions?

Was it cheaper to leave the patient alone -- or did the rehabilitation result in wage earnings, taxpaying and, how about the value to the family who finds father or mother is now no longer chairfast, or legally blind -- or even dead? Where does your gross national product factor that in?

These are but a small sample of the reality. Science does not make medicine cold and technical. It brings change, change that costs money, requires specialists, and improves life.

The world of organ transplantation is only beginning. People will have years added to their lives, good happy years. These procedures will be costly, even in our hypothetical world in which the physicians have fixed salaries. Worthwhile new techniques depend upon physician skill and more physicians to apply it. There are few bargains or shortcuts when one deals with life itself.

Those who condemn medicine as being too technical, cold, impersonal, and that life is maintained when it should not be, could also say that death and disability can be deferred, life can be sweetened, happiness can be bought through scientific advances.

What is the right price tag for such improved medical care? Is not the ultimate base upon which to judge a society the presence of a healthy population? From this comes the other values: shelter, education, civil liberties, security. When we reiterate our founders' premise: life, liberty, and the pursuit of happiness, do these not begin with health? What else should have absolutely first priority for the public's tax money?

The undeniable progress in medical science has not been cheap. It won't be cheap. Adjustments will certainly be made in the physician's fees. Some diagnostic and surgical procedures are too well rewarded. Heresy? No, just the truth. All of the technical procedures have certainly brought ethical and social issues never before faced. Is this the physician's fault? No, it is society's challenge.

Humankind understands that life -- patched, grafted, sewed, medicated, reamed, paced, lifted, augmented, irradiated, transfused life -- whatever medical science can offer, is indeed the ultimate "bottom line." It is the issue which reduces all other problems to trivia. Life is what we have while we are here. It is priceless.

14. No Price Tag

The popular rush in medical care is to contain cost. The fact that our country is spending 14 percent of its money on medical care is cited as a major problem.

Decreasing hospital use has become a prime target.

The cost of medical care inevitably is going to increase. This is not a popular subject. I bring it up, knowing it will be said that I have a bias because I am involved in a factory (medical school) that produces these expensive things called doctors.

If one stands on a high hill, the view is quite clear. One sees a valley in the foreground. That valley is the decrease in cost of medical care in the short range of five or 10 years. It is that valley we are now entering. You might say we are in the "squeezing of the sponge" part of the trip. The sponge has become waterlogged, and wasted dollars are dripping out. Too much hospital use, too many lab tests, too much unneeded high-tech medical care, too many expensive prescription drugs. All that is true. This capping era, corporate medicine fixed-cost-rush we are now into is giving the sponge a series of vigorous squeezes.

We got into this problem because hospitals and doctors were rewarded after the act for whatever actions they had taken. Now we get out of it by placing a premium on frugality of use. That is only the first night of the journey.

The valley has a somewhat gradual slope going in, and we are on that slope now. However, the depth of the valley is not endless. If I may jump around in my similes and metaphors, when the sponge is rung dry a point will be reached, I suggest after a journey of five or 10 years, in which the reality of the next rise will come into view.

I see that very steep rise, here from my view from the hill, and the peak of it is lost in the clouds. I see small markers on it and note a rising GNP percent and then the view is lost in the clouds. Yes, the point for our departure, 14 percent, before we entered the near valley, is but a base camp.

For the truth is we are now watching a transitory event, the wringing out of the over-flush hospitals, excessive things done, mainly because the method of compensation encouraged such acts. I spend no time here on that reality; those things are already part of the errors of the country's history, as were Prohibition, certain wars, the Edsel.

We, however, ignore reality if we think this near valley is the end of the journey. Medical care is not cap-able. Improvements through science and health care are never going to stop nor be denied to those who can benefit from them.

Someone reading this will counter me and say I am ignoring what preventive care will do for us. As we all become believers in low-fat, low-cholesterol, low-sodium, low-blood pressure, tobacco-free lives, we indeed will all be healthier, have less coronary disease, fewer strokes, less lung disease. As we learn to avoid carcinogens, we will benefit.

Such benefits produce a larger burst of people at the elderly end of life. No matter how serene your attitude about such things, the truth is we are all on the waiting list for death. As preventive measures help us pass by the things that took lives in the past, the number of us accumulating at the end, age 75 and up, becomes immense.

The number of very old Americans, 85 and older, is rising three times faster than the rest of the population.

This is why the present valley is but prelude.

A few questions sharpen the truth. Are we going to leave these people in wheelchairs as their hip joints give out? Are they to have a $9 cane, a $40 walker -- or a $3,000 hip-joint replacement and become totally self-sufficient?

Are they to be denied two cataract operations each? Or is semi-blindness more economically sound?

Leave this very old group and turn to the huge numbers who will have coronary occlusion: Are we to deny the validity of an immediate opening of the occluding vessel before heart muscle is lost? As we enthuse over today's cost-containment, where are we budgeting the cost of 24-hour-a-day cardiology teams, able to open the vessels, medically or surgically, and literally salvage the heart? One watches quietly for the politician who will end his career by demanding a capping on this medical advance.

Renal dialysis began as a program to be restricted to those below age 50 -- it is now used at all ages. We speak with enthusiasm of the need to ration such a resource. What politician will vote to deny dialysis to those past sixty-five? Strange, isn't it? Those past 65 do count. They count not only in the values of a compassionate society, they count at the poll. Who will step forward first and restrict cardiac-valve replacement, the use of transplants, the reversal of ventricular tachycardia, the use of the whole range of intensive care and resuscitation?

All those who cried out about the cost of the CAT scanner must realize that such improved technology cannot be denied. The nuclear magnetic-resonance device is another such event. It is but a point on an upward sweeping scale of technology.

For the truth is: life, liberty, and the pursuit of happiness are all conditioned by the ability to enjoy, to have a degree of health. What is wrong with 10 percent of the GNP spent on our health, or 20 percent?

Where is there a logic or rule that can define for an enlightened people the amount they wish to spend on their health and long life?

We are in the valley, squeezing out the things we accumulated in medical costs that were wrong. That rectification is needed. Rising without visible end is the cost of scientific life-giving, life-lengthening medicine. The future of health care is inseparable from the future aspirations of our people.

Living has no price tag. Living with patches, pieces, parts, living where one would have been dead, has no price tag.

15. Compromised Health Care

One must be careful in writing of national health care because it is almost in the same sacrosanct area as religion, abortion, and euthanasia. All are issues so close to personal, internal emotions that one fears to wave a flag in any direction.

Will this country ever develop a planned, logical, coherent health-care system? Does our form of government allow such a thoughtful, reasoned-out cohesive solution? Even with all of the flaws of health care today, and with one political party out in the wilderness looking for a justification to be back in the White House, will the political process still not permit a coordinated plan, a solution? It is not likely.

The reasons are the essence of our political system, a system based upon compromise. Political compromises bring increments of adjustment. These adjustments must find their way between the political realities, the land mines of the power of vested interests.

I do not use the term "vested interests" in a prejudiced sense. National health care is gold-plated, and I mean that in the money sense. When 14 percent of the national treasure is at stake, one is dealing with serious money. Everyone has a vested interest.

All of us recognize the players: the hospitals, the doctors, of course, but it is also critical to recognize the importance of these dollar issues to insurance companies, the pharmaceutical industry, the appliance makers, the entitlement groups. You will note that I did not even mention the patients. What the public really needs will never quite be the issue. What can be done is the reality, not what should be done.

One small sample of this occurred recently. The Department of Veterans Affairs announced that it was opening its hospitals to the general public in certain rural areas where the VA hospitals were underused. The VA sweetened this announcement by declaring their purpose was to "bring quality care to non veterans in remote areas ... "

It does not require deep thought to understand the real issue. The VA Hospital system is overbuilt. Many VA hospitals owe their locations to the strength of Capitol Hill pressures. Demography changes, and some are now in areas where people no longer live. The great mass of World War II veterans is passing away. Vietnam and Desert Storm have not generated enough veteran patients. The clear wisdom of closing the underused hospitals, with huge budget savings, is the answer no bureaucrat, no politician, no lobbyist for the veterans can handle. Open them to the public. Declare it a generosity. Keep the hospitals alive.

Guess who opposes this? The veterans! " ... the plan has caused a furor among veterans who see it as eroding the system's primary mission of serving those who have served their country, and a first step towards transforming the veterans affairs health-care system into a national medical program for the poor." The plan was dropped.

That one example serves as today's lesson. Remember: There will never be a clean, comprehensive health care system in the United States. It will be a compromise: deals, lobby placating, what-can-be-lived-with today, ego-assuaging compromise. Each year there will be manipulations and continuing deals made. The national health care bill of 199X will be a political answer but it will never rest there. It is not because the system is bad or evil. It is because that is what you get when you have a democracy. If you want something different, move.

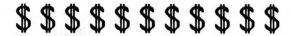

16. Living, Loving, and Dying

We are well into a major change in the American system of medicine. I won't recite all those events, for the reader knows them well. Call it all "corporate medicine."

One of the major questions is the independence of the physician, and the possibility she or he will be forced to make bad medical decisions because the corporate system -- the boss -- will allow economic values to override medical judgments. Don't overlook that issue, it is more important than the question of who pays. Who pays opens the door. Who cares for you is a much more personal action, corporate medicine is not very personal, is it?

The independent, fee-for-service physician, the solo, private physician, the cottage-industry approach, is about to disappear. The last craft is about to undergo the industrial revolution.

The hatmaker, tailor, candlemaker, furniture maker, carriage maker, grocer, each and all have undergone incorporation. Each has been replaced by large stockholding production and distribution systems. And most Americans are satisfied with these changes.

Those urging this process be applied to medicine may be right. I'm optimistic that the impersonality of the corporation, the power of the bottom line, nor the coldness of high-technology medicine can eliminate the ultimate importance of human contact, patient-physician contact. No matter how it is all packaged, computerized, and merchandised, medicine remains different than the incorporation of other services. In the end, it is a form of personal communication.

The English poet W. H. Auden once wrote of this feeling. He said:

> Give me a doctor partridge-plump
> Short in the leg and broad in the rump
> An endomorph with gentle hands
> Who'll never make absurd demands
> That I abandon all my vices
> Nor pull a long face in a crisis,
> But with a twinkle in his eye
> Will tell me that I have to die.

If you will forgive the jar of the last line, a painful honest line, you will agree that Auden is singling out the overriding importance of the human touch. He doesn't ask for the latest technique or laboratory test, he doesn't ask about the cost. He asks for gentleness, understanding, sympathy.

In this era of leaness and fitness, I have trouble with his enthusiasm for a physician that is plump, broad in the rump -- and might have versed my definition this way:

> Give me a doctor lean and keen
> Thoughtful, gentle, never mean
> Give me a doctor who knows
> Life's joys and uncertain woes
> Attends me through test and scans
> Watches for me in the consultants' hands
> And in the end hears me
> When enough I have seen.

I quote Auden and my small addition, for I believe those who are crying out for a cost-effective system are underestimating the powerful value of the healer in any society. No matter what the changes it will not alter the human need for this healing art.

The science of the profession will expand, the economic base will change, but human dependence upon a medical escort through life's troubles will not lessen.

Incorporation may come but, in the end, the bottom line will depend upon the art of medicine. Strange it may sound, the more elaborate the technology, the more refined the methods of profit and loss, the stronger will be the dependence upon the art.

By chance, I was able to see the vast effort made in China under Mao to break the medical profession. The worst of its penalties, punishments, embarrassments in the end were totally defeated, and the profession, the medical profession, was returned to its essential place. The physicians did not force this return -- the people required it.

Living and loving and dying, life is complete in the three. The frightened human needs an understanding guide through the maze of pharmacology, technology, and surgery. Women and men able and willing to carry this duty will always be valued. Needed and valued. Be careful when you make changes.

17. Doc-in-the-Box

One of the clever phrases used in this new era of medicine as clinics pop up in shopping malls is Doc-in-the-Box. I can't hear that pure bit of Americana without smiling. It is such a valid expression of the American scene that my reservations are shattered. I grin, and my imagination takes over. In fact, I can't tell which is imagination and which is reality.

Obviously there are two ways to get medical care at the Doc-in-the-Box: drive-through and counter service.

Drive-through has some real advantages. These are quickness and the fact that you don't have to be attended in the mess and clutter going on inside. You pull up to the large menu board outside which lists complaints and costs: headaches $3; sore throats $3; headache plus sore throat $5.50. Bowels (too much) $1.50; bowels (too little) $1.25, and so on.

One item that sells well is hoku point acupuncture. For hoku, the needle is put in the web of skin between the thumb and index finger. They pop it in at the window where you make your payment and advise you to leave it in for 15 minutes, to keep wiggling and twirling it. You get to keep the needle.

If you want the $18.50 big job, you lean out the window and grasp two metal grips for 15 seconds. At the delivery window, you get the necessary medicines, plus a printout of your blood pressure, temperature, heart rate, electrocardiogram, and your skin impedance. A Coke and a hamburger come with this routinely.

It is all so logical that one can only admire and

envy those who thought it up.

If you want the full menu, you can go inside anytime and order medicine for almost anything: acne, earache, gas, birth control, cough, herpes.

If you have a fever, they offer you a physical examination. This costs $35 if you want a regular doctor to do it, but you can get 25 percent off if an assistant does it.

For a sore throat, headache, and fever, including a nurse's examination, five days of Tylenol and penicillin, hamburger & Coke, it's only $29.95. Careful follow-up has shown that 99.9 percent of customers are fully recovered after five days.

In the unusual case where you really want a history and total physical examination, they have nice booths inside. Colorful curtains give privacy, and they are able to do just about anything.

The doctors who work in this area are skillful and fast. They first get your blood and saliva samples. Then working in teams of three, they divide you up: the top one does head, neck, eyes, ears, mouth, and endoscopy down to the duodenum. The middle man does the heart, lungs, abdomen, using echo equipment. The fellow at the bottom varies the exam depending on the patient's sex. He also uses endoscopy all the way up to the small bowel.

Some places have found it is faster, and the customer likes it better, when they use a moving belt. You undress, put your clothes in a little plastic container, and lie down on the conveyor belt with this container at your feet. They get you through the whole thing on an average of nine minutes.

By the time you are dressed, your printout, medicines, and food are ready. It's like a car wash, and at each step there is a sign flashing, telling you what they are doing. If you want it, they pass you right through a CAT scan.

These places are very ethical. There are some things they just won't touch. They do not do deliveries, and no surgery other than small warts and moles. If your electrocardiogram suggests an infarction, they radio ahead to their emergicenter and by the time you get there, they have angioplasty and streptolysin ready. It is impressive.

One thing people like is the absolute privacy, because Doc-in-the-Box never asks your name and other such things. You pay ahead, and you can either take out malpractice insurance or waive it at your own risk.

You get your hamburger with or without ginseng.

18. Physicians and Politics

My purpose is to foster the merit of politics. Especially the theme that politics and medicine can be, should be, must be, practiced as one.

I didn't know this when I began in medicine 50 years ago. Now I do. Have I changed? Have circumstances changed? A little bit of both.

At perhaps the 99 percent level, new medical graduates know caring for people is what they want to do. The very personal nature of the patient-physician relationship is only complicated by external bureaucracies. Immediately upon becoming a physician, the earliest complications to this caring role -- the patient-physician private contract -- comes from the "outside", from the hospital administration, from insurance companies, from government regulations, from licensing agencies, from a seemingly endless number of interferences. The new physician soon knows that what was to be a noble, contributing way of life becomes one of impediments.

Early on, this external hectoring becomes an enemy, one to be disliked, tolerated, lived with, and to be endured because there is no way to escape. These external forces are labeled as bureaucracy and politics, bureaucrats and politicians. Most of one's career in medicine therefore becomes a matter of the individual physician striving to save, to shelter, the privacy and the quality of the patient-physician relationship against these negative, inescapable burdens.

I knew this well, too, and carried on a private practice of medicine burdened by similar harassments.

After a few years of this, after my share of anger and bitterness over what these "theys" were doing to me; after my share of battles, most lost, with the bureaucracies, a small light began to blink. The light glowed, then burned as I understood what I had not known before and what medical school had not told me: If I wanted to take care of patients my way, I needed to expand my definition of patient care to include influencing the system which was hindering me.

The answer was simple. To educate the "theys" was part of a physician's life. The practice of Medicine was never going to be in a vacuum; it was always going to be a part of the politics of life. Taking care of the sick, the frail, the frightened, and the newborn, the old, the dying, is the highest duty of politics.

Learning that led me to a career which found me often fighting to change a system, to alter what did not seem right, to contest the Establishment. The practice of Medicine and the world in which it is taught and administered are not separate arenas; they are one, and if you, the physician, want what is best for the patient, then you take on the world of politics.

The "theys" become your agents, not your harassers. This was true in my years and now this truth becomes an imperative.

The finest of medical care can only be achieved if the physician is involved, and is heard and seen at all levels of the political system. From department, to hospital, to county medical society, to state and national organizations, to specialty organizations, to compensation and reimbursement, to right-to-life, to right-to-death, to licensing and Board requirements, from the smallest issue to the most exalted, the physician makes the mistake of a lifetime unless he combines duties for the care of the people with the politics of the society in which we live. Every citizen should defend that privilege.

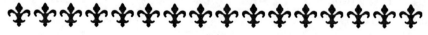

19. The High Road

There are times in the movement of events when all the positioning, talking, criticizing must finally be replaced by action. Such occurs in the small circumstance of one person's tensions with another, on to the corridor whisperings of an organization, to industry moving in on a competitor, to nations seeking war or peace. Now action is happening in that very large system called Medical Care in the United States.

The countdown is on, as the space people say. This circumstance is different, however, from counting down to zero, pressing a button, and causing an irrevocable result. This circumstance of Medical Care also is different than a game in which opponents play, the final gun shot, and the winner has the best score.

What we are all living through is social engineering, an imperfect process that is made more imperfect by the freewheeling nature of the American society. Imperfect it may be, but it is the price we pay for our many freedoms. When the process brings forth a health care system, it will be imperfect, a compromise, the best that could be done working with the system.

What we are experiencing is a living demonstration, a full case history of how our noisy, expensive, unpredictable, biased, litigious system works its way to a solution. Our means of government is very human, imperfect, changing, challenging, filled with checks and balances and compromise. Just what one should hope for in a system "of the people, by the people, for the people."

The process of the altering of the medical care system has now been under way for decades, and the present may seem impossible. Physicians and patients are equally unhappy. For those who are physicians, now is a time of frustration and a feeling that one is but a pawn. Now is not the time to become angry, to let the frustrations cloud your purpose. Now's the time to be the best physician one can be. The physician must not get caught in the commercial network which claims medicine is but another business. The physician must not step one inch outside the role of healer. Physicians are not in this profession for the commerce of it, they are different from industry, business, commercialism, huckstering. They have a privileged purpose, and their task is to prosecute that privileged purpose with all that is good and honorable within them.

My deeply felt message to the physician is: Stay on the high road; from that position you can see the whole scene, and by your conduct make it clear you understand, cherish, and care about the fellow citizens you serve.

Take part in the battle, of course. Give it the best counsel and leadership you have to offer. Be part of the political process. However, always hold your standards above those of others -- all others. Imperfect is this society, and physicians are as full of imperfections as any. Still, the right to serve as confidant to the sick, the worried, the frail, forces one to a path on the high road.

The finally negotiated American medical system is a failure unless it is based upon morality and competence. All other arguments are issues of authority or finance. Place yourself on the higher uncrowded path.

III. ON MEDICAL EDUCATION

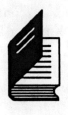

20. On Becoming Civilized

Gate-keepers. Toll-collectors. Standing full in the path leading to the doctor of medicine degree. Part of the obstacle course. Who? What? I refer to the 120, plus or minus, American medical schools continuing to require a full four years of *pre-medical* education before a candidate can even be considered for medical school. A four-year-long gate-keeping-toll-collecting. For what purposes?

Almost any argument on behalf of the four-year "pre-med" limbo fails. If it is claimed that the four years of "pre-med" produce an "educated" person, one need only look at the course content of the majority of "pre-med" students to know there is no time for exposure to "the classics", but instead it is a fight, a race, to get the highest possible grades, especially in the hard science courses, and to get the highest possible score on the medical college aptitude test (MCAT). No matter what the medical school selection committee claims, their eyes gravitate to GPA and MCAT.

The four-year, pre-medical education barrier to entering medical school is a flawed concept, and one that causes more harm than good. All delude themselves who believe the vast majority of pre-medical students can turn away from their overriding obligation to get top grades in hard courses and prepare themselves to make a good grade on the medical college aptitude test. Nothing else counts because nothing else counts as much as getting in medical school.

Claims that this four year hurdle prior to medical school makes for a civilized physician are an example of the dream getting in the way of the reality.

One may be marvelously civilized and still be incompetent. In the most wonderful of all worlds, if one had plenty of money and could relax, play, enjoy four happy college years and know you were guaranteed a place in medical school, then four years at a delightful liberal arts campus, and with trips abroad in summer would, of course, have extraordinary charm -- but that is not what "pre-med" liberal arts education is for 90 percent of those involved. Even if Dad provides you all the needed money, a car, the clothes, the travel -- it looks good on paper -- four wonderful years down at Ole Suwanee -- but it doesn't work out that way. You cannot raise your eyes up to the culture level because biology, comparative anatomy, embryology, physics, chem-1, chem-2, organic, etc. obscure the view. Medical schools make themselves feel "civilized" by urging applicants to have a broad humanities pre-medical school experience. When the decisions are made about whom to admit to the freshman class, the humanities are nice to have, but the grade point average in the "hard" science courses are where the decisions are made. All applicants know that, and freedom to roam through the joy of a liberal curriculum becomes fenced in by reality.

I don't take this stance as a "know nothing" opposed to a liberal education. Why not admit talent to medical school the first year out of high school and let the young person know they are "in" and not at risk -- and get a medical and a humanities education at the same time? Why not? It is possible, we have done it 1600 times. With the maturing experience of seeing the sick, then the exposure to literature, to drama, theater serves to fill in, broaden, explain.

The true liberal education begins with the clinical experiences of medical school, when you see your fellow man up close, and the ultimate reward --

to know yourself -- is superbly facilitated by beginning to understand your own physiology, your own reactions to stress.

Medical school is a liberating education just as much as a liberal education. One of the real benefits of the medical education is to begin understanding the perturbations of one's own heart, digestive system, nervous system, that are brought on by life's stresses. It is wonderfully therapeutic to know that the flipping in your chest is just an extra systole and not important.

Then, most assuredly, once a physician, there comes the ability to travel, to understand geography and history, to learn about cultures, foods, wines, the theater, music, art, to collect, to read for pleasure-- then those things come. Not crammed into four years but for an expanding lifetime.

What pre-medical education did for most of us is that it got us in medical school, and then we on our own, gain our liberal, our humanities education. Competency in helping others comes first, just as knowledge precedes wisdom.

When a colleague tells me that he and his wife spent two months sailing and studying among the Greek Isles, or another took a year to live and practice with the Sioux in the Black Hills of the Dakotas, or another entered Spain at the French border, loaded with reading materials, and spent six weeks working his way with his wife and grown children to Gibraltar, only for the sake of "understanding Spain", and another, only five years out of medical school but now able to take the time and pay for it, spent three weeks on a self-education tour of Southeast Asia -- those are the continuing, completing circumstances which may result in a mature, civilized person.

21. Mirror Mirror on the Wall

In another time and place, I served on the Selection Committee of a medical school for ten years. I was one of the jury that decided who got in the medical school. Ten long years.

A team of three would interview each candidate separately. After the candidate had left the room, the team of three would debate the merits and arrive at a written-down score. Then the assembled full committee would again debate, argue, even trade, and the class was chosen.

All that was long ago, so long ago that I am able to look at the results from a follow-up of 40 years.

From this, what have I learned? Perhaps several things. The overall, even painful conclusion would be that all of our efforts probably made little difference. All of the candidates were intelligent, all had already achieved an academic goal, all had already proved their self-discipline. All felt they had some way to afford the education. All were motivated. We spent hundreds of hours, made thoughtful decisions, and now, looking back four decades later, I doubt very much if the interviews served any real purpose other than this: that in about half of the circumstances we would have been just as well off if we had put in the school those who were rejected. The half we chose would have been found just as well from their written records.

The interviews did serve the purpose of letting three witnesses observe the physical presentation of the applicants and verify deportment, manners, cleanliness. We assured ourselves that we were also evaluating "stability," but that would be hard to defend. I well recall, remember this was in the Fifties, one member of the interview team who had a rule that he would let no one in medical school who had on cuff-links. The interviewer considered cuff-links as a latent manifestation of a gambler. Thus a destiny was decided.

The real value was that the interviews proved to the world that the medical school had scholarly standards, and that was perhaps the principal value of the whole exercise.

During those years, I was a visiting professor in the Netherlands and my education was furthered when I learned that the applicant pool to Dutch medical schools was reduced to a list of names, and that by lottery the names were chosen. The school's attitude was that one got on the applicant list by having met the defined standards and that personal characteristics are essentially unweighable, evaluation by a professor is subject to many variables, and in a true democracy, a lottery was the only honest process.

I am far removed from administration and have zero input into the process for getting into a medical school today. Thus I can say with the assurance that I am influencing no one or any process. Does the selection process miss the point? Instead of making all-wise decisions that are really not that all-wise, should not the same amount of energy and time be used to define to each applicant the expectations of a physician in terms of society's needs, then when the names of all those who are eligible and still want to come are in hand, choose the class by lottery?

Repeated studies have shown that there is no difference in success in a physician's life based upon shades of difference in the applicant's class standing. An excellent study at a Texas medical school has shown that those who were by-passed in the usual process and then put in a school because of a legislative mandate, did just as well as the "carefully" selected. A similar conclusion was reported from

Philadelphia.
    Why not change the orientation? Make it a time to generate in the student and parents an excitement about the value of being a physician, of what society needs and expects--and the value of getting there through your school's program. Why not?

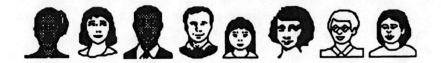

22. Peer Status

Embarrassment before a peer group is perhaps the maximal learning experience. A solo bitter lesson, fully seen by all peers, is the ultimate teacher.

All physicians have similar remembrances. My earliest, very powerful lesson came the day after graduation. I was a one-day old physician.

My medical school class was hurried along because of World War II. We had no vacations; our schedule was 9-9-9-9 (nine months for each academic year). The day one school year ended, the next began. The end of medical school was followed immediately by internship. We finished medical school on Saturday, had Commencement on Sunday, and began our internship on Monday. Medical school offered very little clinical experience. Almost all of the teaching was done by lecture, therefore on Monday morning I put on hospital whites for the first time and reported to the surgical service at 7:00 a.m. for my first rotation. I had been a doctor 24 hours.

The resident told me to do a thoracocentesis, a needle in the chest to take off fluid. I told him I'd never seen nor done one, and he assured me that was why I was an intern and he would stand beside me for the first one. At 7:30 a.m. on day one of my internship, I draped the patient, prepped the skin, was guided into assembling a syringe and needle, aspirated Novocaine into the syringe and infiltrated the skin, then made a tiny stab with the point of the Bard-Parker knife. I assembled the giant, clumsy 50 cc syringe, three-way stop cock, 14-gauge needle and rubber tubing, and with the resident whispering encouragement, stuck in the needle. To my wonder, I began drawing off yellow fluid.

The resident instructed me to take a hemostat, and clamp the needle at the skin margin so that the needle depth would remain fixed and would not inadvertently go too deep or even pop out. With precision and vigor, too much vigor, I snapped the clamp across the shaft of the needle. That is when the real education through embarrassment began.

As the clamp came down on the needle, the needle crumbled in two. The syringe, three-way stop cock, rubber tubing and half the needle rested in my left hand. The clamp fell to the bed, the distal half of the needle teetered in the stab wound for a moment, the patient coughed, and an inch-and-a-half of the 14-gauge needle remnant disappeared into his chest. My patient had an inch and a half long large needle, very sharp on one end and fine steel fragments on the other, in his chest cavity.

At 8:00 a.m., we had a chest film. At 9:00 a.m., we were in surgery, and at 9:30 a.m., the surgeon bowed as he handed me a basin with the retrieved fragment. Before noon of my first day of internship, I had experienced a complete education.

Grand Rounds that Friday featured me on the program, making sure all in the medical center shared my whole story. Grand Rounds means that everyone, students, residents, faculty, nurses, social workers, everyone associated with the medical center, heard every detail about the first patient of my life.

The old adage states it simply, "Experience is the best teacher." When the experience is combined with intense personal embarrassment, the education is not only painful, but forever. Experience hastens wisdom. Embarrassment in front of a peer group sears it in.

Life does not need many migrant-needle moments.

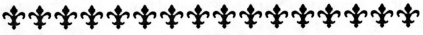

23. Curriculum Packing

I have before me the Minutes of one of the major departments of our medical school and there, moved and seconded, is a motion that pharmacology become an obligatory subject in Year 4 and "that necessary curriculum changes be made to accommodate this." I turned to my files, and there under "Suggested Curriculum Changes," are these gleanings of the School's first 10 years -- formal suggestions, even demands, by faculty:

* "No individual is literate who cannot speak a second language. All medical students must be required to have a minimum of two years of a second foreign language."
* "We are in an era of biophysical-technology explosion. The medical students must be required to have much more physics and biophysics."
* "The physician of tomorrow will be illiterate unless he or she has mastered computer use. We must require proof of computer literacy before graduation."
* "We are not giving students the joy of carrying out fundamental research and carrying it through to a publishable paper. Every student should complete an original research project before graduating."
* "Do you realize that the American population is aging and that the care of the aging is one of the major future needs? Geriatrics must be a required subject for every medical student."
* "Modern physicians have become cold technocrats and have no understanding of the whole patient's well-being. We must teach our students ethics, morality -- and the holisticism of body, mind and spirit."

* "The greatest book ever written is the Bible. No one professing to be a healer should be allowed to leave school without a thorough knowledge of the Bible."

* "The American physician is unable to use the written language. It is wrong for an individual truly "educated" to not be able to compose and communicate in the written language. A basic requirement of the School should be this obligation to demonstrate competency in writing excellent English."

* "You refer to your goal as that of graduating a safe physician. No physician can be safe who is not civilized. The curriculum must include exposure to great ideas, the great men, the great literature of the Western world."

* "How can a physician judge the medical literature unless he knows that which he is reading is reliable? Every student must have a thorough exposure to statistics. One cannot accept medical literature as valid unless one can analyze the statistical method upon which the study was based."

* "The greatest mistake of this era of scientific medicine is that it ignores the overwhelming role of the mind. The curriculum needs much more organized, formal instruction in psychiatry."

* "No student should be allowed to go forward to Year 3 who has not already a firm grasp of biochemistry and physiology. Curriculum time must be found in Years 1 and 2 for much more teaching of these essential subjects."

* "The understanding of people is an essential need of the physician and he must understand psychology -- but before we can teach psychology, the student must take a required course in pre-psychology."

* "One of the greatest ills attacking the whole American Society is poor nutrition. Physicians are not

even taught nutrition in medical school. Every medical school must be required to teach nutrition."

* "Above all, a student must be told how to learn, for it is lifetime learning that will insure the safe physician you speak of. There must be in the curriculum, formal instruction on how to study, how to read an article, how to outline, how to take notes, how to use the library."

* "Sir, I cannot believe that you have a school in which ENT is not a required experience for every student. Do you realize the multiplicity of diseases affecting mankind that involve the ears, nose, and throat? Every student must have a planned exposure to the skills of this essential field."

* "I really do not see how you can allow these young people to go out of here and not have at least some idea about the clotting system. Almost everything that happens to one, whether a stroke, or a heart attack, or a peptic ulcer, involves clotting."

* "Your unwillingness to spend time to understand *Ulysses*, *Finnegan's Wake*, and the seminal work of Proust, D. H. Lawrence, and Kafka is but evidence of why physicians no longer understand patients. From the tragedies and the twisted dramas of mankind developed by these authors one learns about the problems your patients face. It is imperative, Doctor, that the physician learn about the modern world, and what possible better way than through the novelist and playwright?"

Our modern vocal society, with lobbying and confrontational tactics, makes itself heard, and a faculty must fight parliamentary battles, even legal battles to protect the students from increasing demands for pieces of teaching time.

What can a medical school do to satisfy all of these substantial demands for curriculum time or, stated more tellingly, these requests for pieces of the life of each medical student? In its plainest dimension, this issue comes down to how much of a person's life can be used "getting ready." To become a family physician or an internist in a traditional medical school now requires 23 years of obligated "getting ready": primary and secondary school -- 12 years; college -- four years; medical school -- four years; residency -- three years.

The "outsider" may not know this, but the greatest risk to preparing honest, caring physicians is too much curriculum. The threat comes from demands for "obligated" curriculum time. Every hour of obligated or required time takes away the tremendous value of flexibility. Every course forced into the curriculum means that some other opportunity is lost. Every hour of curriculum should face but one critical question: Over the 40 years of this physician's service to mankind, will this exposure help this woman or man to be a self-renewing, trustworthy, compassionate, happy physician?

Note I did not include "learned." For it is obvious that each of his teachers would have had a different interpretation of that condition. Does it mean enjoyment from Dante's *Inferno*, or an awareness of the rhythmic message of Rimsky-Korsakov's *Scheherazade*, or joy in analyzing the play of color and light of a Van Gogh? Does it mean an ability to speak and read Chinese, derive an equation, or discuss the court of the Sun King?

No one living today has the remotest idea what this world will be like in thirty years, yet these young people will be at the peak of their responsibility. No one knows what their world will be, but a faculty can be certain that the ageless values of self-renewal, trustworthiness, compassion -- and personal stability, will still be premier values.

Facts change, theories change. The "hard" data of today is obsolete almost at once. The prescribed literature, art, music of one era may be unappreciated in the next. Even disease changes. The typhoid, polio, syphilis scourges of yesterday are minor issues today. Gentleness, kindness, compassion -- and self renewal, personal happiness and stability -- can we not agree that they are the "hard" curricular obligations? That they are the enduring values by which a faculty must measure its efforts?

24. The Touch of Greatness

Our School of Medicine was host to Dr. Eugene Stead. Dr. Stead is one of the precious achievements of an academic way of life; a scholar and a role model with which the ivory tower of Academe should be peopled. Schooling at any level moves into a high plane of excitement when the student discovers a teacher who is not a warden running a daytime jail, but who is a stimulus.

The painful truth is that one may go to school from kindergarten through college and never have such a relationship. It may all be a sequence of colorless classes, blocks of time spent to get something in the record. When enough A's, B's, C's are in the record, one is finally freed and can get on with real life. So it often happens.

Gene Stead carried the title of chairman of the Department of Medicine at Duke. However, as with truly great teachers, he was always much larger than the title. Often one sees just the opposite, and a substantial title inflates temporarily the occupant up to title-size. Later, when this mantle of authority is lifted, the true smallness of the person is made dramatic by the speed with which his or her influence collapses down to their personal dimension.

Gene Stead serves as an example of the influence a teacher can have upon the achievements of his disciples. It cannot be chance that so many chairmen have come from his followers. Some precious chemistry operates, and those exposed to him took away an aspiration to be like him, certainly the final endorsement of a role model.

An imprecise but accurate word to describe such an individual is "greatness." Greatness is a word that can be tossed around and misapplied until it has no significance. When used in this human endeavor called schooling, greatness becomes the stuff which makes for achievement; the origin of a civilization's elite. To not only tell the student about the importance of commitment, honesty, duty, discipline, but to have them live out the act -- that is greatness.

You must note I did not list in my qualities issuing from a great teacher any applied technology or package of factual knowledge. One can learn a technical trick, a set of facts from a book, a videotape or a lecture, but one needs the exposure to greatness to absorb the unmeasured values: commitment, kindness, honesty, duty, discipline. Someplace, somehow, there is transferred a desire to do one's best for fellow-kind, to do it so well that you too become a leader of women and men.

In our very open society in which everything possible can be printed, filmed, displayed, we have achieved the ability to make someone instantly famous. Fifteen seconds on television can give thief, scoundrel, terrorist, musician, belly dancer, pilot, general, athlete, politician, comedian instant fame. One hundred-thousand fans will fight to gain access to a rock star's or a running back's performance. Fame of this nature can sell jogging shoes, T-shirts, and beer. Such fame makes instant millionaires.

Fame becomes a matter of inches of newsprint, seconds on television and, because of the constancy of need for new faces, our system creates fame daily. Note that the famous are not creating the coverage, instead the media create the famous.

Marshall McLuhan and Andy Warhol squeezed these truths down to two sentences that perhaps will summarize the last 50 years of the 20th century, "The medium is the message," said McLuhan, making clear that television is a device that actually creates its own news. The second of mayhem displayed on prime time becomes the record, and thus totally eliminates the multitude of good and normal events occurring just out of the camera's eye.

Andy Warhol gave the other marker for our times. He predicted that the media have such a vast appetite for fame, for making people instantly well-known, that the end result would be everyone, all of us, could be assured of 15 seconds of fame in our lifetimes.

I belabor fame because one must realize that greatness is a very quiet event and not at all given to publicity. In this field called Medicine there is a fair share of the hucksters, the self-promoters who not only become instantly famous, replete with television interviews, but become rich and popular. If they appeared at our medical schools, the halls and lecture rooms would be lined with palpitating, oohing enthusiasts. That is fame, that is not greatness.

As each class of our students reaches that point of choosing their place for their residencies, the very wise will know that even more important than the choice of city or hospital is the overriding value of gaining access to someone who has the touch of greatness.

There is such a thing as the passing of the torch. The fleeting moment to pick it up depends, to a larger extent than one can realize, upon exposure to its bearer. As the medical graduate leaves school, enthusiastically beginning the residency years, one hopes, wishes they would each have the fun, the reward, the privilege of an exposure to greatness.

An apprenticeship to such a person is the ultimate privilege of schooling.

25. Hunkerin' Down

We were making ward rounds. The resident was a tall, serious, almost silent young man from the High Plains of Kansas. I was on the patient's right, near the head of the bed. The resident was directly opposite, across the bed. The patient's problems were complicated and I was trying hard to draw out the resident and gather him into a two-way conversation. As I have said, he was silent, almost taciturn.

My questions produced monosyllabic responses; his expression did not vary. I decided to ease off further questioning, and tucked my stethoscope into my ears, tilted my head down, closed my eyes, and concentrated on the heart sounds.

After a moment, I raised my head, opened my eyes, and was startled to find the resident's face dropped to the level of the bed. I quickly straightened up and looked over the bed and down at him. He was squatting, sitting on his heels. Rather sharply, I challenged him: "What are you doing?"

Quite calmly, his voice level, he said, "Well, you got me with those questions, and I just hunkered down a moment to think."

Travel educates. One can roam the world, but there is one special breed that hunkers down. Tipping up on both toes, raising the heels, and then dropping the bony haunches down to the heels. Sometimes resting the forearms on the thighs. An ancient Anglo-Saxon derivation somehow brings the word "haunches" through the centuries to "hunkers." A manly manner, a custom seen any place west of Kansas City, from Texas up to western Canada. That's hunkerin' down.

Generally seen in the male species, brought to its best by a campfire and Western boots, hunkerin' down is what one does to facilitate thinking, talking, relaxing, concentration and communication.

My cow-country friend, the resident, had taken up the natural pose of serious men considering a serious problem. In a way I felt complimented, and I was moved to hunker down, too -- but, I realized that with both of us hunkering, and the bed between us, we would not only appear odd to the passerby, but lost to the patient and even obscured from each other.

I stopped our ward rounds, took him by the arm and steered us to the lounge. There we were able to fit ourselves into chairs and get into a serious, useful conversation. He was at ease, and talked out the patient's problem with me. I now understood my friend.

Perhaps ward rounds are not the right scenery, but what this world needs is more hunkerin' down. Summit meetings, international symposia, White House conferences could be considerably improved, even a few eliminated, if there were some honest-to-God forthright, calm, hunkerin' down.

Less show, less press, less ceremonial splendor, less secret and obscured understandings, less performance for the gallery, and more hunkerin' ... that's what we need.

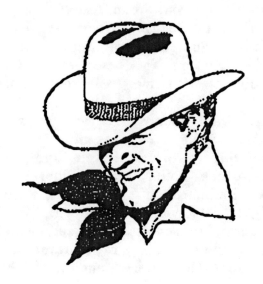

26. Ten Minutes ... Five Words

June! The month of roses, weddings and commencements. All three an unending sequence. Repetition -- but each bud, each bride, each graduate a new, fresh creation.

The roses and weddings are watched over by gardeners and reverends, the commencements by speechmakers.

Honorable, logical, successful people, when commencement speakers become mired in their concern for the importance of their words. Quotations are found, Latin phrases used, references cited, all while the audience fidgets and the dignitary rolls on and on.

After attending commencements for 50 years, even sinking a few myself as the speaker, I have polished a 10-minute presentation that I offer freely for theft, plagiarism, lifting. I don't seek a credit line. This 10 minutes won't hurt anyone, and there are a few who might remember a line or two, a most unusual event for any commencement speech. Perhaps it is not a commencement talk at all -- perhaps it is a definition of living. An epilogue.

Here:

    Your medical school extracts this last ounce of patience from your soul.

    Some total stranger, someone totally unknown to you and of absolutely no importance to your destiny, comes in to tell you about life, to give you a message, to lift you to a greater purpose.

    How can I tell you that you are now

special? You know that. That your role is a precious one? You know that. That you do not have a job, but a calling? You know that. That your role is both minister and healer, that how you conduct yourself is a measure of your quality. You know that.

How can I reduce all of these commencement addresses, given these next several weeks to 16,000 new physicians in 120 medical schools? How can I reduce them all to just a few words, perhaps five words, which you will remember 50 years from now? You may remember them because you will have lived them, because your knowledge being rewarded today will have taken root in the wisdom you will have gleaned.

What five crystalline words?
Five words. Try these:

Live! Let live. Help live.
Try them with me, just five words:
Live! Let live. Help live.
Mull them. Expand them. Turn them. Twist them. Each as a book: **Live!/Let live/Help live.**

The last, **Help live,** is the most earnest injunction one can give you as a physician. It is a definition of your total professional purpose: Helping your fellow man to live.

Everything is expressed: the quality of living, the subordinate, supportive, helping role you must play, not the domineering technocrat, but the sensitive, caring person.

To advise, to strengthen, to help, to cure, to stop short of dominance -- to understand that fine distinction -- that is your privilege.

When your fellow man or woman falters, that is where you stand steady. When your patient improves, don't overestimate your own importance. To know yourself, your limits, your own faults, that is where you begin to ... **help live**.

Never forget that it is life we fight for, not death or some stranded place in between.

Move your mind to the second phrase: **Let live**.

I speak of citizen you, not as a physician, but as a passenger on earth. Learn to let those who are different be different. Don't join the ranks of the "we-they," the haters, the fault-finders. Learn as fast as you can that others have different religions, religions which serve them well, different customs, languages, foods, clothing. However, learn well that they have the same gamut of emotions you do, they live out their lives seeking just about what you seek. They laugh and cry and hurt in the same way you do. Grow wise enough to know that the other person is entitled to his or her way. You may not like it, but be large enough to comprehend it.

Tolerance is not cowardice, but is a measure of one's own size.

Let live.

And the final word: ... **Live!**.
Ah, there is the primary book.
Help live is the professional you.
Let live is society's you.
Live! (yes, with an exclamation point) is you.

Grab your diploma and **live!**. Extract every honest and honorable joy you can out of this life. Think of this life of yours as your single reason for taking up space on earth. Use your time and space with every bit of exuberance you can muster. Crank up every unit of energy, ambition, motivation within you and **live!**. Live full blast. Get involved. Do. Care. Work. Give. Sample. Taste. Test. Travel. Inhale. Explore. Know. See. Hear. Influence. Challenge. Be. Be worthy of the time and place you have been given.

You are on this stage for an unpredictable length of time. The curtain will fall assuredly. Give the performance of your life -- **Live!**

I am done. We will not meet again. Your life will be led in a world I will not know -- a simple truth measured by the calendar. We have had a brief 10 minutes together and I have offered you five words.

Oh my physicians, my sisters and brothers, go from here and then ..
Live!
Let live.
Help live.

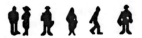

IV. LESSONS FROM LIFE

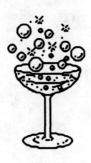

27. Lessons from Shortstop

This is a story dealing with education, and the power of experience. Lessons learned through living take time; for all of us, time runs out before we have learned enough. Learning that time is life is one great leap towards wisdom. Carelessness with time is self-destruction.

I report on such a lesson which saved for me an enormous amount of time. Remember, time is life. From this single experience I learned that I did not like baseball, could not play first-class baseball, and that I should use my time for things I could do.

I also had my first ineluctable lesson that all men are not created equal. Our great founding document may claim this is true, but from experience, bitter experience, I know that to not be true, at least for baseball.

Beginning young, I played baseball -- morning, noon, and night. Played catch, hit flies, shagged balls, played move-up, bounced a ball off the garage door, oiled my glove, got shoes with spikes -- got ready. When old enough for American Legion baseball, I was there. Made the team.

For three summers I was the first baseman. Between playing, daydreaming, talking, oiling my glove, and bouncing a ball off the garage door, I did little else. Time is life. Time, life, and baseball became synonymous.

In the third year, the year I was 15, I quit baseball. I never oiled my glove again, or bounced anything off the garage wall.

The reason is simple: I learned through experience that all men are not created equal. That summer Billy moved to town. He showed up one day at practice and stood around; he finally asked if he could try out for shortstop.

Our coach scratched and stalled because he was faced with a problem. We were an all-white team, and no black had ever been on the team. No black had ever asked. Billy was in old Keds; the rest of us wore splendid spikes. His glove was a miserable rag; ours were oiled and ready.

Coach stalled and thought, but finally, in the fifth inning of the practice game, told Billy to take over at shortstop.

Billy was different. He poured across space with fluid ease. When a ball came to his area, there was a blur, the movement not broken into a jump, or a twist, or a turn, but a liquid, melted action. This part of the performance I could admire. It was when from this whirling image the ball shot out like a white dart to first base, that I became personally educated. The ball came at a speed not characteristic of our American Legion level. The ball flashed toward me, and I was still moving my glove toward it when it struck me in the stomach. The pain was made worse by the roaring laughter of my teammates.

We finished the game, I survived, and survival was in question. I found myself praying that no one would hit to Billy. I was a man before a firing squad. He would move to his right, to his left, then with no hesitation, no change of stride, no visible cocking of his arm, the white bullet flashed to first base, dead center on my belly button.

We were not born equal. He could get a ball to first base faster than my reflexes could respond. If I played on a team with eight men of similar skill, I could be killed.

Experience delivered its lesson. There are true baseball athletes and there are others who know the rules but don't have the ability.

I staggered through a few more games, dreading every game, and my only sympathy came from the man who had been our shortstop. He suffered the hurt of losing his position, but he was lucky. At least he was not risking his life. We both took up golf.

The time saved has been a treasure. I have never played again; never been to a game, can't stand it on television, don't know any of the players. Billy was a memorable teacher.

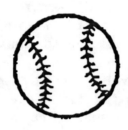

28. Peaches Ellis

Experience encompasses knowledge, training, book learning, teaching, and of course, living, especially the value of having done something at least once before.

These portentous words lead to my message about experience and how painful it can be to acquire it. Part of the pain comes from the vulnerability you have at that very moment of gaining the first exposure. If the event was a success, there is a glow, a warmth which fixes that savored moment in the bank of felicitous memories.

However, if that moment of gaining experience is a disaster, and you learn by the error, not by the victory, then burned into your soul forever is the pain, embarrassment, humiliation -- the awfulness of the lesson. Assuredly the lesson is learned forever.

As does everyone, I have an ample supply of what one may call "learning by bitterness," any one incident which, when recalled, makes my ears burn, my pulse quicken, and causes a fleeting grimace. A very simple example defines the power of this "learning by burning."

My position on the high school football team was right end. My best friend was the left end, and there were no fancy complications such as offensive team, defensive team, and special teams. If you were on the team, you played the whole game.

We played regional high schools, our home games were played to a full stadium, and the big Thanksgiving Day game was played before 25,000 people -- quite a stress-producing big moment for young players. Being on the team was a big event, and there was a considerable amount of ego inflation which transferred the stress into cockiness.

Our Terre Haute team played in such famous places as Sullivan, Linton, Clinton, Brazil, Crawfordsville, and even Indianapolis. The game I describe was played in Georgetown, Ill., a town of very modest circumstance -- so modest that we considered ourselves the sophisticated hot shots from the big city, Terre Haute. I don't believe there was any grandstand or bleachers, just a hundred or two Georgetown boosters on the sidelines.

We had heard that Georgetown had a small fastback named Peaches Ellis, and we had come to Georgetown committed to show Peaches Ellis how football was played in the big league.

Georgetown had the ball, and on the first play a halfback came sweeping around my side of the line. I gave him a bone-crushing tackle behind the line of scrimmage. I got back on my feet, looked around for some compliments, and discovered that Peaches Ellis had run 80 yards for a touchdown. I had tackled the wrong man. Peaches had executed the perfect hidden-ball trick. The only encouraging part of it was to learn that my best friend, the left end, had tackled the other back who had come around his end, all hunched over a ball which was not there. The crowd of 200 hooted, jeered, and chanted, "Peaches! Peaches! Who's got the ball!"

At half time, our coach was livid. He gave us hell and ranted at what an embarrassment we were. He kicked benches, snarled.

The afternoon got worse. Seldom did any of us tackle the right man, certainly not Peaches Ellis. The Georgetown coach had a series of hidden-ball, end-around, last-moment laterals which our team had never seen, been coached in, nor imagined. Peaches Ellis was the shiftiest, quickest little magician imaginable, and the only times I tackled him were when he didn't have the ball.

We lost, and the trip home was somber, the bus silent. The coach hunched down alone in the seat behind the driver. A bunch of 17 year olds slumped in their seats, egos bruised, filled with doubt and feeling miserable. Our only comfort was the relief that girlfriends, classmates, parents had not been there. One's peer world is very small at that age.

I was much older and had lived and hurt quite a bit before I understood who had failed in Georgetown.

We weren't the ones for whom the lesson was fire in the soul. There was only one person on the bus who was deep in personal failure. Only one who knew that poor coaching, poor performance at half-time, poor performance now in the bus when these kids needed solace and leadership, that he was the inadequate piece. Our coach had had the real lesson. We made the mistakes, but he was the one who had put us out there without a fair warning. He was not man enough, mature enough, to provide leadership. At half-time, at the end of the game, now on the bus, he could not get beyond himself and give the words of reassurance we all needed. He had failed.

Many times in my teaching and physician life, I have reminded myself that one cannot teach all of the variables and one can't avoid some mistakes. One cannot make all illnesses go away and some things can only end in loss. That is where leadership, physicianship, not bits of information about technique, must take over. Being able to rise up, pull the students together, to pull the patient and his family together, to laugh, cry, to go on -- together. Within every loss there is some kind of victory, even if it is only in remembering the other days. Our coach didn't know that.

29. Moral: Beware of Greed

My family's home, during my ages of 15 to 18, was near a public golf course where one could play all day for 25 cents. This bargain was irresistible, and summer was devoted to golf.

Logically, this should have led to an enthusiasm for the game which carried on through adult life. In fact, the last time I was on a golf course was in high school.

One problem was temptation: all the golf you could play for a quarter. I readily got in 36 holes a day. Then 45 -- and my bargain-hunting made me push for 54 holes a day. To reach this number, it was impossible to play with others; I could not hold to the pace if I played in a twosome or a foursome. I kept increasing the rate at which I moved (remember, this was before golf carts), and I finally was trotting to the next lie of the ball. The results were measured by the number of holes played, not by the score.

The golf bag made trotting difficult, and all the clubs were an unnecessary burden. In the last year I played, I streamlined the game to a level of efficiency and carried a two-iron and a putter only, no bag. Starting at daylight, running between strokes, and playing alone, I could comfortably get in 54 holes a day. All for a quarter.

One day on hole 3, a 125-yard hole, I topped the ball with the two-iron and it trickled the entire length of the fairway on the ground and into the cup -- a hole-in-one. A hole-in-one from a flubbed shot. I was playing alone, but a couple was allowing me to play through and witnessed it for me. I won a $5 gift certificate to Montgomery Ward for this feat. All for a quarter.

Few people have played golf in this manner, and therefore do not recognize what an improved sport it becomes. The quick tempo of my game made the normal, mannerly foursome confining, tedious. I found only one partner who fully enjoyed the modified game. He was Vic, a high-school classmate, and he had my same enthusiasm for the speeded-up sport. He later became a very successful lawyer.

The speed of my game was a joy, but there was one burden I could not break. The explanation for my retirement at age 18, and one understandable by any golfer, is that I developed a tremendous hook which I could not shake. A hook rolls well and it was not a bad handicap for my game of speed golf. That is the reason I never tried any instruction or tutoring. I gradually adapted a useful stance and stood at a 90-degree angle from the fairway, aiming straight off in the wrong direction, right angles to the cup. I struck the ball, it zoomed up and away, and then began a great graceful curve back towards the logical fairway. If the direction of the cup was south, I gave the ball a great blast to the west.

This performance was greeted with loud cheers of derision. Anyone playing on the next fairway was frightened by the confusing stance of this eccentric golfer and assumed they were under fire. I finally solved the hook; I quit.

Although I have never again played a game of golf, I stopped at a driving range years later, stepped up and blasted off a drive. The ball whirled up, beautifully, powerfully, then came the bending to the left. On and on it sailed, off course, finally disappearing over the left-hand safety net.

The hook had survived the years. The hook was a kindness, for without it, I perhaps would have persisted at "speed golf", and society would have not been gentle. Up to age 18, it is called youthful exuberance but there would be low tolerance for a middle aged sprinter hurrying his way through foursomes. Before you laugh, remember, I once made a hole-in-one.

30. Tabasco Sauce and Ice-Cold Beer

An engaging attitude for living is expressed in the words: "Try everything ... in moderation." This sentiment, at least for public consumption, should include the caution, "if it is legal."

Legalness is interpreted with a broadminded latitude. No rule is perfect; all rules need to be tested and, on occasion, if not broken, at least well bent. The idea of trying something at least once is just about the same thing as "growing up." Growing up is the prime time for trying a bit of everything. Trying enough things gives one a menu for what one wants to do, or not to do, with the rest of life. Too many people grow up too much under the "Don't do it!" rule. They later suffer from a middle-age agitation, realize how much they have missed, try to catch up, and end up making a botch of their senior years.

One of the valuable things about the junior years is that you can make mistakes which are covered by the useful excuse, "Oh, he is just growing up." If one waits until the senior years to sow a few senior oats, then the rumor mill quickly is bruited about that "that old goat is getting senile."

Our rule for living begins to get clogged with modifying clauses: Try everything, in moderation -- if it is legal -- if you don't get caught -- if you are the right age -- if you are in the right place -- if it doesn't embarrass your children -- if your mom can stand it.

A moment of reflecting on our extended rule reminds one that we have left out another injunction: " ... as long as it does not risk your health." Even a brief exposure to Russian roulette may cut off further adventures.

One recalls examples of trying everything. One of my high school friends sought to impress his peers with his capacity for spicy foods. He up-ended one of those ubiquitous bottles of Tabasco sauce and made clear his derring-do: he it drank it all down. We were all impressed, he proved that he lived the rule, "try everything." He forgot "in moderation." He impressed all of us for about five minutes. Then came his pain, agitation and vomiting. He eventually recovered. He later became a hospital administrator, probably knowing he had already experienced hell.

Another example: In college there was a Golden Gloves event, and one very aggressive young man in the heavyweight class announced he was going to win the match with his very first blow. He rushed from his corner, swung a masterful roundhouse right, missed his opponent by a large distance. The powerful swing met no obstacle, and his humerus head slipped out of the glenoid fossa, dislocating his right arm at the shoulder. He was assisted from the ring, defeated by an opponent who had not struck a blow. He too had ignored the basic rule: "Everything in moderation."

He later became a mortician and, to our knowledge, never again struck a blow.

Another example: A bar nearby our medical school served frosted mugs, 12 ounces each, of ice-cold beer. An enthusiast, caught up in a variation of chug-a-lug, quaffed 10 full mugs in rather short order. Intoxicated? Perhaps, but the immediate problem was hypothermia, violent shaking chills, inability to speak because of clinched jaws. "In moderation?" Hardly. "Legal?" Probably. "Harmful to health?" Acutely. For the long range, it may have been therapeutic; he never drank beer again. He became a very conservative internist.

These youthful indiscretions are offered only to

show there are intelligent limits to our aphorism. One may add the rider, "within the limits of good sense." I cite them also to make the point that all three of these foolish acts in youth gave no clue as to the adult who would come out.

With all of those shadows on our rule, it still is a bit of wisdom. To expand one's experience, to travel to out-of-the-way places, to try the unknown moment, to take on the challenge not before met -- or, as has been said -- "live dangerously, as carefully as possible," is how life should be used. Even though most such experiences come in the early years, one should not interpret such advice as counseling a later life of boredom. Even the most successful of careers needs right-angle turns. What one does well and repeatedly can soon become a rut. Don't let our modified aphorism push you into a life of boredom. Surprise yourself, surprise all those who have you "figured out." Break the bonds. Plan your career so there are periodic times for recharging, learning anew, finding yourself and your family again. Be predictably unpredictable. Of course, within legal limits, moral limits, health limits, financial limits, responsible limits, etc., etc., etc.

31. On Building Character

For a year and a half, between ending high school and going to college, I drove a truck. I can report that truck driving is a very strong stimulus for higher education. Pre-med, medical school, and residency all had their moments of exhaustion, but they were minor compared to pounding the highways long before freeways. For a non-union driver, the loading and unloading of a 10-ton semi-trailer were additional dividends of inspiration, each dividend delivered in a single 70-pound cardboard carton.

For those who press weights for joy, the thought of lifting 70 pounds may seem a mere snap of a bicep. When placed in context, and context is a warehouse in Atlanta, Georgia, the unloading dock is on the sunny side, and you have driven all night and half the day to get 10 tons of load to that sun-scorched furnace at 2 p.m., you have a context worth study and analysis.

A 70-pound cardboard carton moved one time is do-able, but even then it is a strain. No handles, no rope, instead a smooth, undentable, ungrippable cardboard carton.

Ten tons is 20,000 pounds, and the mathematics, although simple, has a deep, lasting impact on mind, body, and spirit: The 280 individual 70 pound box physical acts require stomping up the truck ramp into the breathless caldron, reaching up or reaching down (each equally wrenching), clasping the solid, smooth cardboard mass to the chest, staggering back out a full 40 feet into the warehouse to your ever higher mass of identical boxes.

Today when my friends tell me of their inner ecstasy, some use the expression a "high", that intense physical exertion gives, and seem critical of my inactivity, I dream away for a moment and recapture the total, absolute sunk exhaustion of the truck days.

It may seem that this was a character-building experience, not an ordeal, but an opportunity to test and find oneself, and from such testing came the iron of maturity. I can report that such an ordeal has nothing to do with character, nothing to do with the nobility of labor. Sweat is sweat, hard work done under miserable circumstances to make a living is hard work done under miserable circumstances.

My response to eager believers of the virtue of desperate physical labor is that they must try it sometime. For me it had motivational value, straightforward motivation towards getting away from, out of, that form of work which utilized the human body as a work animal. Nothing done in loading or unloading that mammoth truck required any quality above that which a trained chimp could have done -- could have done better with a box under each arm.

The motivational value had nothing, zero, to do with the beauty of testing the body, of the purity of sweat, of spiritual invigoration set in motion by good, honest labor. The value was directly related to the thought that never left me: "I am doing this job because I need the money; so help me, I'm going to spend the rest of my life using the part of my body that a machine or chimp cannot offer; from here on, it is going to be an intellectual adventure."

An intellectual adventure is what life can and should be. It is in our capacity for higher planes of thinking, of imagining, of creating, of caring that we find justification for being. Chimps, machines, and now computers have their roles, but when one moves beyond the loading and unloading of 70-pound boxes, on beyond pulling barges, moving stone to build pyramids and great walls, toting cotton, digging ditches, one moves on to a level of freedom.

That freedom becomes worthless, or less valued, or falsely gained, unless it is replaced by a willingness to use, use to exhaustion, those qualities which are uniquely human, of intelligence, caring, hoping, creating, weeping, consoling, remembering, reading, writing, healing.

Human intelligence opens the whole world to us, but we remain small, menial, still just a body to be hired, unless we reach out with those abilities which are the special privilege of humankind, to lift, to carry forward, to sustain, to support, not boxes, but those we serve.

32. Knowing When to Cut

I recounted the motivational value of truck driving. My truck driving days were interrupted by days back at the plant. The truck sat idle until sufficient orders had been written by salesmen to justify a whole truckload for Dallas, Atlanta, Chicago, Los Angeles, Indianapolis, or other regional bases. The plant manager, a black-browed, frowning, joy-free man who announced his rank by wearing a hat at all times, would seize me by my belt and put me in an assembly line when there was not a truckload ready to go.

These lines were moving conveyors upon which empty bottles were put at one end, and 70-pound sealed boxes appeared at the other end. In between, the bottles were filled, capped, labeled, and packed. The velocity with which the belt moved determined everyone's degree of commitment -- and when in high gear, it was a formidable experience. What I carried in the truck was glue, paste, ink, white shoe polish, and wallpaper cleaner. That is what these assembly lines were bottling.

Any idea you have of happy employees gaily chatting as they sat doing their simple task needs to be replaced with a line of grim, intense people, eyes and hands flicking at top speed, every nerve concentrating to keep up with the unyielding moving belt.

The heart of each line was the large vat of mucilage, paste, ink, or white shoe polish. Beneath the vat was a horizontal wheel, fitted with slots shaped to hold firmly the bottle. With a clickity-clack rhythm, this wheel rotated one slot at a time clockwise; when the slot had advanced, a signal neatly opened a valve and allowed a metered, two, four, or six ounces of mucilage, paste, ink, or white shoe polish to spill down into the bottle.

This was the moment of truth, if one may borrow a phrase from Hemingway's bull. When the slot advanced, the valve opened, the liquid poured -- bottle or no bottle. The destiny of this entire factory went to pot in a moment if there was no bottle in the slot. The mucilage, paste, ink, or white shoe polish spilled onto the moving belt, the belt moved forward carrying a thin layer of disaster. The entire line shut down, everything had to be disassembled and cleaned -- a project which took time, time which became large when you knew everyone's quota and possible bonus were at stake; time which became unbearable if it happened twice.

Driving the truck on the open road seemed almost an escape compared to that awful instant when your hand fumbled and the bottle did not slip into the slot on the wheel. The valve opened and the substantial squirt splattered on the moving belt, you pressed the emergency button to stop the whole line, and struggled to smile and encourage sympathy from the line workers glowering on your right and left.

White shoe polish has a special quality of persistence which made its spillage larger than the novice can comprehend. There is something about it which makes it seem to grow. If you spill four ounces of white shoe polish and then add a gallon of water to wash it away, you suddenly have a gallon of white shoe polish. Deep in its nature is the ability to increase, to permeate, to stain white forever. It grows like a monster, coming to life and escaping, not eating all in its path, but marking their clothes, their hands, where they touch their faces, their shoes, their footprints, until white spreads over the whole factory.

A spill of white shoe polish meant instantly to all in the line that there would be no bonus for the day's work. Factory workers do not take such events lightly, nor do they write petitions. Instead, they become abusive, in profane, uncomplicated terms.

The manager seized my belt and, cursing at a very high level of communication, marched and shuffled me into a new assignment having to do with unloading the box cars which brought raw materials to the plants, such as flour, the basis for making the paste and wallpaper cleanser. It came in 200 pound bags.

Wallpaper cleanser is an unknown substance to my children, but there was a time, especially in the era of soft coal for home heating, when a part of spring home cleaning required the use of wallpaper cleanser on the interior walls of the entire house.

This material was a quite pleasant, nice-scented, doughy mass, not at all unlike Play-Doh. It was packed in a can, a pound to the can, and to open a can, blop out the pink, rubbery, perfumed contents, knead it in your hands, and begin rubbing the sooty walls was a satisfying experience.

At the factory it was the company's premier product, and the man who presided over the feeding of the wallpaper can had the premier job. There were no bottles, no liquids, no spills; instead the drama was in a large, grinding machine which took all of the ingredients into its maw, and at the far end sent out a continuous, unending, unstopped 4-inch wide column of wallpaper cleanser, steaming hot.

It was a massive toothpaste tube, with a giant compressing it at a constant rate, and instead of a quarter-inch-wide round column of Crest, there came a 4-inch wide perfect column of wallpaper cleanser. There stood the hero of the factory, a good-looking man in bib overalls, always starched and clean. In his left hand he held an empty can, in his right, a gleaming butcher knife. He thrust the can against the nozzle, held it firm against the pressure of the cleanser avalanche, and at just the right moment, just when the can held one pound of cleanser, just when it was full and a lid could be sealed on, he gave one great whack, clean and lovely, with his butcher knife, slicing the pink rope through. Down went his left hand, putting the filled can on the conveyor belt, back up it swept with an empty can, captured the inch of cleanser already bulging forth, pressed it until the can was exactly full, whack went the knife, sliced through was the cleanser, and on and on he went, never making an error, never letting the giant pink column squirt loose on the floor, never filling the can beyond capacity, never under-filling. He was the hero of the plant. He had an important job, he did it well, he was admired, respected, compensated, and he was proud of his achievement.

One could elaborate on the honest values represented here of a person doing the right thing in the right way in the right place, and how this is all that life and happiness can hope to be.

I don't miss the lesson and I accept it as the truth. That is a lesson as it is directly observed. I want to go a step in a different direction and make a stand for the metaphor he was demonstrating. Above all else, he stays in my hall of memories as the ultimate example of knowing when to cut, when the act is long enough, when the container is full, when the experience is not too little or too much. To know when it is time to make a clean, ending cut and move on to a new filling.

Stretching a point? Too grand a metaphor for a too simple event? Perhaps so, but for me, the image that remains is of that very happy, competent, confident man in bib overalls, controlling his events and knowing when it was just enough.

For life must be that way, and one must

recognize that there are chapters, phases, units which make up one's career, and there are circumstances when it is critical to know when the chapter is full and done and it's time for a clean cut. The lesson cannot be learned too soon: to compartmentalize, to have a life of chapters, phases, units, to sense when each of these is complete unto itself and to make the clean cut. The path will be full of those who hang on too long, those who won't risk a new scene, those who dangle.

Go on by those people, make fresh turns, find new adventures, new challenges. Learn to cut when the experience has stopped using fully the best you have to give.

33. Poll Taking on Hospital Hill

Legend has it that Kansas City takes its name from Kansas, the bordering state. Kansas takes it name from the Kansa Indians. Their name is derived from the Indian word *kansa*, meaning southwind. True or not, it should be. No one who lives out in the Great Plains or here in the adjacent areas, can hide from the constant wind from the southwest.

It moans through the eaves, tilts the trees in a permanent northeast slant, brings in over this region a steady delivery of dust and pollen. It provided the basic blowing for the sweeping away of Dorothy to the Land of Oz. It is a formidable force, leaning forever on those plants, animals, buildings, and people in its path.

With this climate fact in mind, I need to introduce another geographic circumstance. Southwest of my house runs a certain length of Main Street. This particular area has become well-known as Fast Food Alley. Cheek-to-jowl, superburger-to-taco, colorful franchises have lined themselves like glass beads on a necklace, each bead a different design and color. How do they all make a living? Can there be so many unusual ways to produce the same food in 60 seconds?

Now, it may be only a touch of paranoia but, right or wrong, here is my observation. Any contrary evidence will not be fairly heard. The combination of the unceasing, unyielding *kansa*, the southwind, these sources of styrofoam packages, cups, paper bags and napkins, plus the inbred diet of medical students, leads to a paper-plastic alley extending from Main Street to my front yard. My house is at the end of this alley, and east, north, and west of my front yard, the ground drops off sharply.

Some specific act of thermal physics turns this southwest wind into a whirling dervish that dances exactly at the apex of 25th and Holmes, at *Diastole*. The whipped weathervane on my roof cannot cipher this williwaw and simply rattles in agitation. The high walls and somewhat odd shape of my house act as an enticement, a trap taking grand amounts of fast-food debris out of this whirlwind. If the city wants to economize on street cleaning, it can simply send one man with a plastic bag, a big one, to my front gate. Nature will deliver to him a rich harvest of the best trash of Fast Food Alley.

One always tries to turn bad into good. This whirlicane which has chosen to perform on my doorstep is a challenge. How to make use of it?

Time will provide other answers, but for now the answer is poll-taking. Companies pay out large sums of money to learn where their product fails or succeeds. Who buys it, and what layer of society? What a plum it would be if McDonald's knew whether the debris in my front yard was in its favor. To know medical and dental students spread your debris in a ratio of 2-1 over your nearest competitor could be precious knowledge.

There is an additional debris poll I am taking that is not related to the southwind. At least not likely. This has to do with the heavier items of bottles and cans. These come at the rate of six a day, and evidently are dropped at the site of their becoming empty. That seems reasonable -- my paranoia has not reached the point where I assume citizens are driving deliberately to my house to toss their empties. I think this unusual collection is related to my location near the city hospital emergency room. Here are the facts: Budweiser cans and bottles lead handily. Half-pint bottles of Gordon's Gin and Canadian Club have a dominant position. Wine? Pint bottles empty of muscatel and port are the winners.

If anyone can think of any solution that can turn a small profit, I would be very interested.

34. Gardening in the City

High on lists of therapeutic lifestyles is tilling the good earth. Getting down on the knees, eye-to-eye with a weed, then wrenching it from the ground does the soul more good than Valium.

A sundown stroll along the rose bed, sniffing and admiring, gives the day's problems a glorious answer.

Such pleasures are a reward of suburban and country living. However, fate took its turn, and my time for gardening places me deep in this mid-America city. In fact, my garden is not only in the Heart of America, as Kansas City likes to be known, but is in the inner-city.

The country gardener warms his tales with stories of fox, possum, and raccoon visitors. These little moments with the wild are not exactly part of city gardening. True, my walnut tree has a lively squirrel trade, and occasionally a rabbit will burst from under a juniper. The animal that brings uniqueness to city gardening is Man. No fox, no geese, just Man.

When your garden is an action spot such as this, tilling and toiling are different. A weed is still a weed, the roses still need spraying, the bagworms still prosper, but that is where stillness ends; serenity is not guaranteed.

When Friday at five comes, there is an hour-and-a-half roar from Thank-God-It's-Fridayers across the street at the tavern. Then, as if a clap of thunder scattered them for shelter, all scurry away -- scurry to their suburbs and their tidy golf courses, gardens, and games. All is peaceful about my inner city garden. For awhile. Then begin the first sirens of the ambulances bringing in the weekend casualties. My garden is next door to the emergency room of our hospital.

From all points of the compass, the wrecked, wrenched, stabbed, and shot get hurried past my garden. I can stand among the hollyhocks and hear the sirens singing, hurrying for the Emergency Room. Then come the flashing lights past my corner as ambulances and police cars whoop it up.

City gardening, of course, is not all different from country gardening. It is still a matter of digging, composting, feeding, watering, and weeding. Yet there are certain adventures that one might miss with rural gardening.

When I was more of a novice, I planted 100 hyacinths along the street thinking their color would bring a new joy to the tired neighborhood. I walked down along Holmes Street to admire them, and a nice car pulled up, an attractive young lady with a shovel and bucket popped out, and with energy began digging up my plants. When I somewhat urgently urged her to leave them alone, she pushed the shovel in with increased vigor and advised me to go away. She added that this was abandoned property and that she was simply trying to save the plants.

The idea that my garden was abandoned had not occurred to me, but I took this as a serious criticism and worked a whole Saturday afternoon to put in 10 quite handsome Alberta Spruce trees. I thought these specimens would assure the passerby that the garden had an owner. The next morning, I walked out to the stone wall, enjoying the thought of seeing the results of my Saturday planting. All 10 trees were gone. Between 6 p.m. Saturday and 8 a.m. Sunday, my trees had been given a new home.

In the city garden, Man can appear with just as much surprise as does Brer Rabbit in the country. Last spring, I found a sleeping bag, very wet, tattered, and dirty among the rose hedge. It seemed abandoned, and I tossed it.

Two days later while I was weeding near the hedge, a bottom in ragged trousers came backing out. I raised my hoe in self defense, just as I remembered Mr. MacGregor did in the briar patch. The trousers rose from their knees and, with pleasant good cheer, a quite seedy man asked if I had seen his sleeping bag. He told me he'd been living under the bridge, had cracked his hand, "Me and my buddy was playin' around," and they had staggered their way to the Emergency Room. When they told him he had to stay overnight, he explained, "Me and my buddy jes' put my stuff here in the bushes."

Staggering visitors are fairly common about my garden. I am evidently on a direct path between their watering hole and a halfway house. Weekends seem to take a toll on the halfway-house patrons. Seeing me spading provokes memories of their good days down on the farm, and almost each weekend brings through my garden some gregarious, wobbling, slightly beery fellow, always pleasant and anxious to tell me about Pappy and brother Billy Joe and how it was down in Texas on the farm.

There is a corner in my garden, nestled around with deep rose hedge, and there I have put a swing. Strategically, carefully put so one can sit there, gently swinging and see nothing but the trees, bushes, shrubs, roses, peonies. See nothing but green growing things, Sit there moving, almost floating, back and forth. You can watch the robins scouting for worms, see the cardinals flit their color, scratch MaMa-HuHu's ears, and then, like a distant trumpet, comes the first clear call of the evening's first ambulance.

The city's music begins. Man is in the garden.

35. The Battlefield

On ward rounds in a city hospital one can be an impressive diagnostician by demonstrating the value of observation. Old and new scars, crooked fingers, tattoos, dental care, sunburn, calluses, worn shoe, nicotine stain, hair, skin, hands, nails: the road map of life's trip, the wear and tear.

One of the young doctors commented that such visible findings were only because of the hard-used social class seen in a big-city hospital. I more or less agreed with him, but later was mulling over another piece of protoplasm with which I am familiar -- mine.

I came up with this personal scoreboard.

The scar	How I got it
two inch smallpox vaccination	doctor created, plus infection
three pock scars, forehead	measles
two inch scar, inside left arm	bicycle accident
one inch scar, point of chin	tripped running to first base; first base was a rock
one inch scar, left eyebrow	fist fight
bent index finger, right hand	baseball
scar, crescent shaped, roof of mouth, hard palate	fellow stuck open hand in my mouth while

The scar	How I got it
	playing football. Finger nail stuck in roof of mouth
very fine white scar, right side of chin	mole removed
scar, bridge of nose	boxing
scar, thin and white, right upper lip	sparring match, boxing
bent fourth metacarpal, right hand	street fighting
scar, back of neck	boil lanced in medical school
surgical scar, left knee	removal of ruptured medial meniscus, torn in high school, completed in beach volley ball
surgical scar, back	removal ruptured disc. Fell, hiking in Italian Alps.
long jagged scar, back of right hand	ripped hand on metal patio chair when my tethered dog (tethered to my wrist) lunged at another dog

I have to admit the story is not very glamorous and would make a poor film script, but it is my own evidence of having been alive. I rather enjoyed making the inventory.

This personal battlefield is essentially a tally of an American boyhood through the 1920s and 1930s, with a few evidences of later life, too.

I try to recall the character-building, true-blue ethics involved in the various sports; but frankly, I can't. Most of the scars of life don't show. Most of the scars -- and rewards -- are deep, inside, and private. Cuts and scratches give not even a hint of the true bruises and pain.

36. This is Liberation?

During one of the very peak periods of what I thought was a busy career, I had the good fortune to have an immensely able secretary. She handled every detail: appointments, phone calls, billings, correspondence, diplomacy, filing, travel. In every way, she was leaned upon, put upon, requested, used -- and did it all perfectly. Someone once said that if you really want to get something done, then go to the most successful man you know. His secretary can get it done. This lady was exactly that person.

As I write, I note that I readily said, in defining a successful person that "it" would be a "he." And of course the image of the secretary would automatically be that of a "she." That is the way it was then.

With that bow to the changing scene, let me get on with my theme.

During this busy chapter, I one day gallantly commented to the secretary, "I'll bet you will remember this as the busiest time of your life, and when you are married you will breathe a sigh of relief."

She did marry, to my shock, and moved half way across the country. Five years later we met. She was the mother of three children, her husband a successful physician.

In a spirit of remembering the old days, and our shared vigorous work, I said, "Well, it must be a relief to be out of all that which you went through. Those were terribly demanding years and I remember how harassed and tired you sometimes felt. At least you now have the busiest years of your life behind you."

She didn't even look up. She simply said, "I didn't know what busy was until I had three babies quickly, was running the entire home, trying to be doctor's wife, housekeeper, mother. What we did back then was nothing compared to being a mother."

That lesson has stayed with me, and as I watch our medical school graduate class after class of women physicians, and as I follow their lives and see them handling career, home, marriage, pregnancy, AND children, I am in full awe of what they are putting through.

This may be titled the era of "women's lib" but it just is not. This present change in our social roles is working only because women are doubling and tripling their responsibility. The satisfaction in seeing my profession become half men and half women is balanced by my awareness that these women are carrying mental, physical, and emotional loads that a man cannot understand, nor, of course, ever will.

37. Tourist Class

You step up to the airline counter and the attendant smiles at you, a zipping, on-and-off facial action. Tapping her computer, eyes never again in your direction, she produces in you a moment of agitation when she "can't find you" in the computer. A few more pecks corrects the spelling of your name, and you exhale with relief. The monster agrees you exist.

Then, in rapid order, the attendant fires a series of questions, never glancing at you. She asks the questions a thousand times a day. You hear enough to guess her intent, and somehow say yes or no in the right sequence: confirming your destination, you have one suitcase, you want to check it, you want an aisle seat.

She taps the gadget, it clicks and ratchets and agrees that all of these things are acceptable. You hand over your luggage, go through a security checkpoint, again have a moment of agitation when the tunnel's loud buzz announces to all your possible guilt. You empty your pockets, go through again, and the machine gives you a green-light endorsement.

You stumble your way onto the plane and work your way through the first-class cabin. Damn! How can that scrawny kid afford a first-class ticket? Look at that fat toad in a yellow-and-green plaid suit traveling on his expense account. Having champagne in a stemmed glass. The attendants scurry you through this green pasture.

Hundreds of traveling sheep are herded into the aft cabin. The same quick facial tic of a smile is applied by the flight attendant who then does her joyless mission. Up and down the narrow aisle, rapidly, repeatedly, asking all in an expression-free voice if they want coffeeteamilkorsoftdrink. Dyawannabyadrinkfertwodollars.

The tiny trays of food are rushed down the aisles, the crowded masses of prisoners are in their seats, eager to erupt into the aisle.

At your destination, you exit through the forward cabin and again feel hostility toward those fat-cats who had been in these wide seats with their silverware and cloth napkins.

You all gather at the carousel and begin the Russian roulette game of hoping your luggage has come. Tons of bags spill out on the wheel. Again, your anxiety level rises. It finally all comes out well. You and your bag meet and then, the unexpected reward. There is justice under heaven. That yellow-and-green plaid expense account irritant from the first-class section lost his luggage. All is good again. Democracy has proved itself.

You stagger away with your bag to the rent-a-car counter. There is a bored young woman behind the computer. She gives you the facial movement smile, stabs the computer, and the same monotone begins: a series of questions not really spoken, not really heard. A final dit-dit from the computer and you are approved.

You go to the curb to get the rental car bus and arrive in time to see a wonderfully long, sleek, six-door black Mercedes limousine and a large posterior covered in green-and-yellow plaid stepping into it.

How can a mature man, a man of infinite wisdom and experience, a healer and advisor to the ill, hate someone he never saw before? Is this physician still unfinished? Has he not learned to love all mankind? Evidently, there are still a few flaws to be worked on.

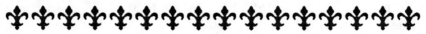

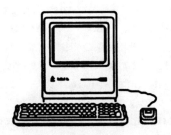

38. Friendship

In late September 1946, I was in a jeep just a block from the Kabuki Theater in Tokyo. My driver asked if I was thirsty, and we pulled to a stop in the middle of an empty cross-section. One lonely Japanese taxi was stopped there, and its driver was busily tossing wood into the stove in the trunk of the cab. With his wood-burning engine refueled, he chugged away, smelling like an American barbecue.

My driver and I took our tin cups, and from the large Lister bag that was suspended from the temporary trellis in the middle of the cross-section, we had our fill of heavily chlorinated water. Every neighborhood had its suspended Lister bag, the single dependable source of water.

We had driven that day from the waterfront of Yokohama to Tokyo, and with few exceptions, no factories were standing, only occasional black chimneys belonging to the destroyed buildings.

We drove on past the Kabuki Theater, turned left a few blocks later, and there, white and unharmed, stood the quite lovely St. Luke's Hospital. Like the emperor's palace and all of Kyoto, this missionary hospital carefully had been spared the bombing that had removed all of the industrial areas of Yokohama and Tokyo. Now the hospital was the 42nd General Hospital, a tertiary care hospital for the entire Far East Command, and my home. I was the cardiologist, young, unfinished, enthusiastic, and thoroughly overworked.

That untouched white island, a first-class hospital, was not only the main referral hospital for American personnel in Japan but for Shanghai, Saipan, Okinawa, Korea, an oasis of modern medicine.

Last year, I again was driven from Yokohama to

Tokyo, an agitated scene of explosion, not of bombs, but of buildings, freeways, express trains, people, cars, trucks -- an explosion of prosperity. I left the taxi at the front door of the Kabuki Theater and winnowed my way through the masses of people to the intersection where had hung the Lister bag.

The movement, the hurry, the energy of that intersection was exciting, almost humorous. Charlie Chaplin's *Modern Times* was being lived out. There was a logic, but the overall impression was of a small, black-haired, well-dressed multitude of wound-up dolls, careening about with purpose, avoiding darting spotless taxis, each with white-gloved drivers. Could this be where we had sat on the hood of the jeep, had our drink of water, and watched the sooty driver stoking the stove of that single, lonely cab?

I walked on down to St. Luke's Hospital, which I found still handsome. I went down to the heart station where I had had a Sanborn electrocardiograph as my sole equipment and read 50 electrocardiograms a day. Now it was a marvel of computers, technicolor echocardiograms, and great, silent robots passing patients through scanners and magnetic fields.

When I was the cardiologist there, my technician was a tiny Japanese physician who, upon the surrender of Japan, had been assigned to this role with the American army. We worked together daily for more than a year with never a moment of conflict -- or conversation. He was quick, precise, silent. Yet from that strange, uncommunicative time we found something, if not a friendship, perhaps an understanding of trust and respect.

Through the 40 years, our New Year's greeting cards had been exchanged, always formal, never with extra message. Never had he asked for a favor. Now, today, I was to meet him as his guest at the revolving restaurant atop one of Tokyo's many splendid hotels.

I came off the elevator not knowing exactly what to expect. There he was, a man in his sixties, the same slender wisp, a tense, silent man, moving with the same little fluttery manner. A hand shake with the intensity of two butterflies.

We went to our table and had two hours together, no reminiscences, no "Do you remember?" No laughter. One question. One answer. Next question, next answer. He was the host, and had already selected the menu. Attentive waiters scurried about, and my anticipation was of an elegant Japanese meal. A silver wine chiller with a bottle of French champagne appeared.

Then with a flourish the waiter placed before us our entrees, with silver coverings. Simultaneously, two waiters whisked off the cover dishes. There was our main course: bacon, lettuce, and tomato sandwich on toast. My moment of disbelief passed, and I smiled, he smiled, we raised our glasses to each other, to our memories. No words.

I slowly ate my BLT and savored the thoughtful effort he had made in selecting for us what he knew was a great American delicacy. We silently ate, sipping the iced Mumms. He asked about my children, I asked about his. East met West.

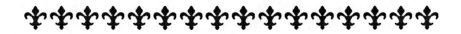

39. Father John

Father John Lerhinan died in November 1987. He was my best friend of my adult years. He was that special value often found missing in a physician's life: an access to the world other than medicine.

I speak of the role, of the value, of one or two friends from whom you never asked, never gave, never took anything remotely material. Of a friend or two who were not a part of the ambitions, the politics, the frustrations of your professional career; of a friendship so very distinct from those important relationships one has with colleagues or partners. A quite different emotion than that of love or romance or passion -- but a vital human experience: a friendship. Yes, this is an essay on friendship -- sustaining, lasting, trusting friendship.

Where fits Father John?

When the Second World War ended, a large new American experience began. Armies of Occupation were sent to Germany and Japan. An Army of Occupation was a second society moving into, on, a native society, and it involved setting up a complete functioning bit of America. The occupied nation, exhausted, bombed, decimated, had small resources upon which to rebuild itself, yet the occupying army had the right, the right of power, to take any home, building, facility, and food it required.

The strategic bombing which destroyed most of Yokohama and Tokyo had purposefully preserved specific structures from destruction. A handsome, modern hospital, built by the Episcopalians before the war, had been spared by the bombings. It became the 42nd General Hospital and was the only general hospital for the American military forces.

This Episcopalian facility for prosecuting their missionary effort was a most unusual, handsome physical structure. The center of the building was a cathedral, with its ceiling soaring up in the finest English tradition; the ground floor had the usual church format, and could easily seat several hundred. Surrounding this cathedral on three sides was the hospital.

A relationship had been established to the hospital making use of the church's high, vaulted ceiling: rising for five floors like a series of balconies at the opera, each patient floor extended out into the church, an area spacious enough to easily accommodate wheelchairs and even beds. Thus, each floor was both hospital and cathedral.

The sense of soaring sanctuary was increased by the use of leaded blue stained glass and deep-blue tiles. When the American army took over the facility, we added a new complexity, a complexity that would have surprised and horrified the original designers. The Sunday religious services were expanded into three faiths. The Episcopalian service was incorporated into a good, utilitarian, single Protestant service. Then, in a matter of minutes, a new group of worshipers moved in, not only on the chapel floor, but were brought in at each of the balconies, and suddenly the church was a synagogue, and a rabbi chaplain took over.

When his service ended, there was another scurrying around of arrangements at the altar. In a twinkling, the Catholic chaplain, robed, and supported by acolytes and altar boys -- usually enlisted men from the hospital technicians -- held Mass. Above, beds and wheelchairs moving out, new ones moving in through the five floors of the cathedral-*cum*-hospital.

The hospital was a full general hospital, complete with surgery, orthopaedics, obstetrics, pediatrics, medicine -- everything. In addition, it was not only the hospital for the American military in Japan, but also for the increasing number of civilians coming to participate in the complexity of the Occupation. Economists, lawyers, engineers, businessmen, Red Cross workers, wives, dependents, in addition to military personnel, were all patients in the hospital. Because the chapel was intact, not destroyed as were the other churches of Tokyo, and was such a handsome building, the allied forces and families living in Tokyo came for the religious services.

My office was on the second floor, immediately adjacent to the chapel balcony, and Sunday-morning patient rounds had to be adjusted to a coming-and-going and catch-the-patient-as-you-can style. As patients came and went to one of the triad of services; I found it best to simply go to all three of the church services and quietly move among my patients, whispering a question, checking a pulse, hearing a complaint.

Chaplain John Lerhinan, Captain, was the Catholic priest assigned to the 42nd General Hospital. Tall, 6'-3," trim, pink-faced -- a face that glowed with a smile -- sandy-haired, in uniform, as were all of us, except when in robes for Mass, a voice that moved in mellow brightness with an up-and-down cadence, and with a little mixture of Irish and New York State accent.

Lunch followed the three services, and Father John and I usually ate together. His typical opening remark was, "Well, how did I do today? Did you feel an urge to come forward?" Wit and good humor were quick and he brightened his basic scholar's approach. Conversation with him was a series of questions, never too personal, but each carefully crafted to require a blend of thoughtful answer. Our friendship began there continued over a 40-year period.

The 42nd General Hospital was a very civilized,

well-run facility. The officers had a private dining room, starched tablecloths, flowered centerpieces. The service, by tiny, kimonoed Japanese girls, was meticulous. At the end of the day we adjourned to our club, complete with orchestra, pool, and excellent food. Father John enjoyed people, and of course, never was flirtatious, but at ease with the nurses who were also officers.

John was not chaplain to the officers only. The largest part of his flock was among the enlisted men. When he first arrived at this 42nd General Hospital, he had rationed his time so he alternated evenings at the enlisted men's club and the officers' club. Soon he realized that his presence at a Saturday night blast at either place was inhibiting, and he developed his "early fade" approach -- smiling, chatting, weaving among the crowd, quietly moving, never saying good-bye as he cheerfully managed his successful escape: "I vanished among the angels!"

As a chaplain, he enjoyed a benefit that physicians did not have, a car. Doctors could summon transportation from the hospital motor pool, and a driver would take us on errands. But Father John, because of the need to visit widely over his Tokyo parish, had the most precious privilege, the privilege each of us missed most, his own personal jeep, driven by himself and, an unlimited gasoline supply.

His Sundays were his workdays, as he called them; Saturdays were for exploring. From Kamakura to Nikko to Fuji, and all over Yokohama and Tokyo, we could roam. Between his explanations of priestly duties, and mine justifying medical needs, we calmed all military police and explored freely.

Our time in Japan ended, and we went our separate ways. He began moving up through the ranks of his religious order, the Redemptorists. I started up the path of academic medicine. His responsibilities moved him into increasing demand for travel, inspection, teaching in the affairs of his order, and my path was equally one of travel, inspections, and teaching. We met in Boston, in New York, Washington, Los Angeles, London, Kansas City, and then, when he moved to a very high position in Rome, we had delightful times there.

Never, in the whole 40 years, while together did either of us tell a joke, have more than a beer or two, play at any game or sport, discuss women, sin, confession, damnation, or the Bible. Yet, in person and on the phone, we had essentially a nonstop conversation. Interruptions of a year or two were not noticed, the conversation with ease picked up as if it had never stopped.

He was from a large Irish Catholic family, educated in the parish schools, and from the earliest age was planning for priesthood. He was a booky and shy young boy, and went on to get his doctorate in economics at the Catholic University in Washington.

I was an only child from a Southern, areligious family, schooled in public schools, with all the enthusiasms for sports and girls that one is supposed to have, and with a medical degree from a Midwestern state university. None of these differences interfered with our pleasure of each other's company. Instead, our differences in background, schooling, profession seemed to disappear, replaced by lively, enthusiastic conversation.

I told him on one occasion that my real purpose in our association was to find out where all the Buddhists, Muslims, and other faiths spent eternity if they couldn't get in a Catholic heaven, and his response was, "Oh, they're up there, all right, we rent them space."

Building on his education as a doctor in

economics, he became a very knowledgeable investor, and with seniority, he took over the management of a substantial portfolio of his order. He was very successful in this, and to my remark that this was an unpredictable chapter in the life of a hard-working priest I had known in Tokyo, he replied, "It just shows what good living, prayer, and good friends on Wall Street can do."

He loved the great stone churches, loved them for their beauty and for their strength and statement of permanence. When we would drive by a particular Redemptorist cathedral on Broadway in Kansas City, he would nod sagely and mutter, " ... fine piece of real estate."

He was intrigued by my China experience, and we talked after each trip about his church in China. I told him of meeting a roomful of Chinese seminary students, and he wryly observed, "The way things are going, we will need those priests, we can't find men now. The Holy Roman Church perhaps will have to insert the word Chinese into its title."

At the end of 40 years, we met to celebrate. He came to Kansas City, announced he had investigated the restaurants, and was going to host our dinner. As always, we talked broadly about the world, about personalities, about books, about politics, about large things and very little things.

After our dinner on that last visit of his to Kansas City, we walked up from Crown Center to my house. As we strolled up the hill, we chatted, and then suddenly he stopped and turned and pointed to the top of the Hyatt hotel and said, a bit breathlessly, "Say! That is really a tall building!"

I glanced at him, and I realized he was having angina, and was using the old subterfuge of distracting attention while he rested. Twice more, we stopped on our way home.

Before we parted, I said, "John, let's find out about your angina?" He laughed and turned away my question, "I promise you I'll give up butter. Look! I've led such a pure life there's nothing else to give up!" We laughed, shook hands, slowly, firmly, and with not another word said, we exactly knew.

Ten days later, I was telephoned from his office. He had died suddenly. Yet a friendship of the quality I am describing does not end. Almost daily, I will have a small chuckle over a remembered remark, or, for a fleeting instant will anticipate sharing a well-done book.

Such friendships are not sudden, but must be worked at, cultivated, renewed. Old wood, leather, metals are similar: all age well and respond to gentle polishing, to use, to time. One must make an investment or two in this special vineyard of Friendship.

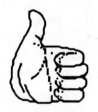

40. Me and My Shadow

A young man, age 32, with notebook, ballpoint pen, and tape recorder, came to see me. His purpose was "to get the story" of the School of Medicine. It certainly has been told often enough, but for him, it was something new.

He was a bright, perceptive young man, but I was not prepared for his opening statement. Leaning over his recorder, pressing the right pair of buttons, he sat back expectantly and encouraged me, lowering his voice to a more mature, resonating note, and said, "Sir, now that you are in the shadows of your life, it perhaps is appropriate to sum up what you have done and what regrets you have."

The recorder purred along, he sat with his pen poised, alert, pleasantly expectant. I nodded sagely, cautioning myself it would be ill-received if I leaned across the small table, seized his necktie and, while choking him, explained that no man should open an interview with such an alienation of interpersonal relations. What an opening! "Shadows of your life... "

Instead, my mind enjoyed a full right and left split, a dichotomy. Part of my thinking apparatus moved along with his questions, trying not only to answer but to educate; to let him lead with his questions but to give answers that would teach him, to take him from his nice naivete to a level of useful sophistication.

He did not know that my mind was chiefly having a delightful time being 29 years old again, standing in Dr. Paul Dudley White's office in Boston, in Massachusetts General Hospital, drinking sherry. Yes, the tape recorder can verify that I did not accuse the young man of ageism, did not tell him of the merits of things learned after age 32, and that my responses to him were better than I would have given 40 years earlier.

The tape recorder cannot produce any evidence to show that I was in Boston, it was 1948, and a lovely day with sunlight streaming in the small windows of the old building. We were there on that day for what we young people thought was a sad moment. The sherry was for our toast to Paul Dudley White as he shut down his career at Massachusetts General Hospital, avoiding mandatory retirement, and moving his office to Beacon Street. All of us recognized this was the end of an era, the end of the "PDW" influence in Cardiology, and we were the last Fellows he would ever train. We felt it could not be a more saddened event, and we Fellows moved rather ponderously and piously about the room, attempting to reassure the senior staff and especially Dr. White, that his life had been well spent.

I gathered up my own glass and came up to Dr. White, managing that smile one features to prove braveness at hopeless moments. I wished him well and, encouragingly, suggested now that he was retiring he could write his autobiography. Quick, oh so quick and bright and exactly honest, Dr. White laughed and said, "Oh really? I'd always planned to do that when I was old. There is still so much to do! Retiring? Hardly!"

I retreated across the room to my colleagues, men equally unfinished, equally convinced that age 62 was near-senility. I reported my conversation and we enjoyed our shared joke about the old chief who didn't understand that he was a fossil.

Twenty-five years later, when the invitation came to me from the Chinese to inspect their health care system, that same Paul White, age 85, flew straight through from Boston to Hong Kong, rested one night, the next day entered China with me for a physical ordeal: morning, noon and night; left China without even stopping in Hong Kong, flew directly to Rome to see the Pope, and then back to Boston to pick up his office appointments.

The "little old man," age 62, who I had so lugubriously retired in 1948 had 25 and a half years of vigorous life after our glass of sherry. Write an autobiography at 62? Why the story is just beginning! In the shadows of one's life? One has been tested, the lessons have been taken, the fires of spring replaced by a steadier flame, the goals are now focused, shaped by altruism and knowing what is possible. In the shadows? Only if one seeks them.

How very much alive he was at 85, and how painfully little I had understood at 29. When we made our trip into China, he was still so very much the man he had been. All that had happened in 23 years was that I had become 52, and moderately mature. The reporter knew none of this.

V. HOBBIES AND INTERESTS

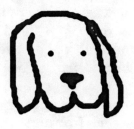

41. MaMa is a He

Although I own 2501 Holmes Street and am legally the laird, the true possessor is my big black dog, MaMa-HuHu. No phone call is complete, nor any letter, nor visit, without the specific question , "How is MaMa?" It is obvious to me that it is his house and I work for him.

He recently had surgery, and he received six cards, two floral arrangements, and an emergency phone call from Vienna. Against all rules, he one time crossed the busy street. I had two phone calls criticizing my inattention and a police car drove up with MaMa in the back seat. The policeman criticized me also.

When my mother was heavy with child (I like that phrase, it has a frontier, old-days ring), she bought a dog so that upon my arrival I would have an immediate constant companion. This plan was successful, and now, decades and dogs later, I can't imagine life without a doggy buddy. Hair, fleas, itch, rug spots, pained endings I have had fully, but the good times have been the remembrance, the other things just a small token, fare for the trip.

Girl dogs, boy dogs, little dogs (twin Chihuahua sisters), big dogs, happy dogs, grumpy dogs, social dogs, finicky dogs. Bullies, cowards, clowns, loafers -- I have lived with them all and we have had good times together. When the time happens as it does, and my house is without a dog, I develop a strange emptiness, a restlessness begins that is made worse by returning home and not having the need to "put the dog out."

Getting up in the morning is incomplete without a head to pat. The day is hollow, it echos, something is missing. The water dish sits empty for days, finished with its importance, then the brush, the leash, the flea powder, water dish, go to the back of the cupboard. Time goes by and I find myself staring at my bookshelves, then I reach out and pull down my copy of *Dogs of the World*. I have begun my private search committee. The next hairy companion is but a matter of time.

Eight years ago, Amigo, my German shepherd, died, and my period of reconciliation took almost a year -- reconciliation with the fact that life was no fun without a dog. I warned myself that this next one was perhaps the last dog I would have and, that I wanted something special.

Gradually I narrowed the search to a handful of breeds, a Weimaraner, a Rhodesian Ridgeback, a Rottweiler -- and then I was in Bellagio, Italy and saw a handsome giant of a dog -- huge, sturdy, alert, dignified, well-mannered. His feet and legs were like heavy staffs. When I somewhat hesitantly patted him, his chest thumped like a drum. Tail and ears cropped, head held high, this big fellow was a dog among dogs!

I learned he was a Giant Schnauzer and when I returned home I hurried to get reading material. Purebred dogs are different from humans. We humans come with a whole alphabet soup of genes. We have no constancy of pedigree and the result is the wonderfulness of our variations. The effort to explain us has resulted in livelihoods for psychiatrists, sociologists, and psychologists.

A pedigreed dog has all the limits and all the security that comes from stereotyping. A cute, bouncy, animated, alert, intelligent Chihuahua is what you know you will get when you get a Chihuahua. A Doberman, a German shepherd, a Dalmatian? All predictable. All dogs I have enjoyed.

Now I was eager for my first Giant Schnauzer. I

joined the Giant Schnauzer Club and got their monthly magazines. I read *Dog World* and finally found a breeder in Canada. We agreed that the next male was to be sent to Kansas City at age 10 weeks. The book said he would grow up to be a lovable, dependable clown, and that he would require great affection and would be a natural guard dog. I learned that his appetite would be intimidating and his energy unbelievable.

I had been making trips to China and learned a delightful expression: "mama-huhu." That is the Chinese way of replying to the question of "How are things?" The phrase is used as our "Oh, just so-so." Or one could say, "Oh, a little of this, a little of that." The Chinese have considerably embellished this thought but have kept the same meaning, and their reply tells you, "Oh, okay, just as usual, horses and tigers." In other words, a little of this, a little of that. MaMa means horses. HuHu means tigers. MaMa-HuHu therefore says quite nicely things are the same as always, just the usual number of horses and tigers.

When my dog arrived, he was 12 pounds of black, roly-poly hair, tumbling and stumbling over his big feet. I knew he would grow up to be huge, a horse, so I called him MaMa-HuHu, and MaMa is a he. MaMa does not mean Her Her. It means Horses. And he is a He.

He did grow up. And up. He now is a mass of 110 pounds that quite contentedly sits in anyone's lap. He is an impressive professional at his guard-dog duty, yet has never even remotely nipped, bitten, or had an unpredictable moment. He is devoted to women, and has no resistance to them. I mean human women, not Schnauzer women. Men require longer to get on his acceptance list.

His appetite did prove impressive, and 18 cups of dog chow is his daily snack. He swims vigorously, loves to retrieve in the surf, and sits on top of the sprinkler. He cannot tell a flower from a weed, and his big feet press all equally. A good snowstorm brings joy to him, and when it is 10 below zero he rushes about snapping at flakes, eating the snow, rolling on his back in the deepest drift. A freezing rain doesn't penetrate his deep coat and, as his eyebrows and whiskers freeze up, he becomes a glittering horse-tiger.

His method of attack is interesting because he uses his huge body to knock the opponent down. Some place, tucked away, is the original set of genes constructed to make his ancestors the guard dog in medieval Munich, and he takes that role most seriously.

Hundreds of years ago, someone set out to create a great, strong dog able to weather any climate, able to pull loads in the day and patrol the grounds at night. MaMa doesn't know this is what he was bred to do, yet the purity of pedigree has him fully prepared.

Recently, when he had surgery, the veterinarian's assistant telephoned and said, "I am calling about MaMa. She is ready to come home." I didn't tell MaMa about the pronoun. He's very sensitive.

♂ ♂ ♂ ♂

42. Chance? Fate?

"Chance is a fool's name for Fate."

Here is the test of the aphorism. And, another chapter in life with my dog friends.

On Wednesday night, May 5, I put the two dogs out for their last run. Twin brothers, year-old black Miniature Schnauzers. MaMa-HuHu's successors. After 15 minutes, I called for them to come in. No dogs. Stood up on the stone wall, whistled, yelled, "Wei! Ni Hao!" ("Hello! How are you!" in Chinese.) Tried my best enticement: "You want something good?!" Always works. They know they get a treat. But no dogs.

I put on decent clothes, got in the car, drove the neighborhood. Yelling, whistling, clapping my hands. Saw a police car, asked, no help. Returned home, again went to the back stone wall and yelled and whistled into the night. Again got the car and drove a complete circle, two blocks in each direction, windows down, whistling, calling, "Wei -- Ni Hao." No dogs.

Kept this up until 1:00 a.m. Raining. Searched the yard again. To bed. Worried, but still thought that with their halters and name tags, someone had picked them up to protect them. Probably a neighbor who would call in the morning. But no dogs on their side of my bed.

Next morning, got up at 6:15 and drove the neighborhood all the way to Gillham, to one block east of Troost, to the railroad on the north, to 29th Street on the south. Raining. Relieved not to see two little black lumps beside the busy roads.

Waited by the phone for message that someone had found them. No calls. Called lost dogs agency;

called the vet who has their number registered. No dogs.

    At 11 a.m., gave up. No phone call had come. Would put ad in paper. Probably someone had dognapped them for a reward. Drove in the rain to main post office to mail each daughter a package. Crossed four roads with heavy, speeding traffic. A busy half-mile of city traffic. Left post office to drive down Main Street to buy gasoline. Down Main Street between Crown Center and world war memorial area. Never drive in that area. Used this route only because I wanted to stop at the cleaners. By chance, glanced up on west side, my right. In bushes distinctly saw a small black dog with a red halter. Absolutely was Ni Hao. About 8 feet up, above a stone wall. His head was turning quickly. He was looking east. No more than one second before I passed. Was it imagination?

    Traffic very heavy. No parking area. Drove to entrance of Penn Valley Park; stopped just off Main Street. Parked car and trotted back to area, whistling, calling out. No Ni Hao. Of course I had seen him. Or had I? Followed along the muddy path just above a stone wall for a hundred yards. Wei! Ni Hao! Wei! Dog or aberration? Wish replacing fact? Drove up onto level of war monument; Put windows down. Drove along, whistling, yelling, "Wei! Ni Hao!" And their most tempting call (always gets them a dog biscuit), "Want something good?!"

    Saw a bearded man, long sideburns, black leather vest with steel studs, bare chest. He waved a large chain at me and scowled an invitation. Remembered this was an alternative lifestyle area and they were misunderstanding this white-haired man who had all windows down, was whistling, yelling out, "Wei, Ni Hao!" "Want something good!" Beat hasty retreat. No dogs.

    Parked car in front of old St. Mary's Hospital.

Took umbrella and walked two blocks along bushes on terrace, near Main Street, east and below the war memorial. Calling, whistling. Had I really seen Ni Hao? Yes, of course I had. I was not cracking up. I knew my phone number. I knew my date of birth. I almost knew my Social Security number. It was a reality, not an apparition.

One hundred yards, 200 yards. No dogs. Three hundred yards, suddenly an excited little, dirty, muddy Ni Hao rushed up to me, leaping and yipping. Grabbed him. He wiggled and squeaked. Still no Wei.

Whistling, calling out, "Wei!" Looked across deep grass, up a slope. Saw little, exhausted Wei. Unable to go further. No tail wiggle. Limping. Ni Hao, excited, jumping about. Picked up Wei, who was a limp rag, head hanging down. Checked Wei. No cuts, no broken bones. Simply exhausted and chilled.

Carried both dogs, umbrella, in rain to car. Put them in back seat. Took two wet dirty, bedraggled, burred Miniature Schnauzers home. Each got a dog biscuit. Drank and ate. Ate and drank. They curled together like two pretzels. Went to sleep.

"Chance is a fool's name for Fate."

43. Mississippi Yellow Ear Retires

On April 9, at 10:00 a.m., in the Los Angeles airport, the portly lady peering into the X-ray viewer gave a grunt, muttered a command, and my briefcase was set aside for inspection. The attendant popped opened the bag, dug out my electric razor, my tape recorder, and then, with sheer, lovely, utter disbelief, came up with a very large, angry turtle.

It took quite awhile to satisfy everyone that the turtle was not a cleverly disguised bomb. Finally he was back in the briefcase, then beneath my seat on the plane, and away we flew to Hawaii.

Mr. Turtle was, as were others in the friendly skies of United, on his way to retirement on the beaches of Hawaii.

What brought him to this grand evening time in the sunset? It is a long story.

Life has moments of occasion. Births, graduations, marriages, retirements are life's milestones -- rites of passage, rites of spring, rites achieved.

My house recently experienced one of those moments, moments somehow blended by the sadness of time passing and a reaching for the next experience. Mr. Turtle retired.

It all began in Washington in the spring of 1968. Lark, age 15, Lea, age 10, and Pop went down Wisconsin Ave. to McCrory's Five & Ten store in search of a pet for our new home. After some consultation, the girls invested 25 cents each and got two quite small turtles, each smaller than the diameter of the quarter they cost.

I read that the chances for survival for home-raised turtles were small, that they usually died of infection, and even gave infection to the owners. So for a year they were kept in the small aquarium with streptomycin in the water, and each day antibiotic drops put in their eyes.

In 1969 they survived the transfer to Kansas City and then followed eight years at the Ward Parkway house, summers in the lily pond, and winters in a steadily enlarging aquarium. They were also steadily enlarging, putting away an ounce of raw liver twice a week.

The equipment grew: larger filters, ultraviolet lights, heaters, rock platforms for sunning. One experiment ended quickly, enthusiastically. We added some goldfish to the aquarium to give it some life and color. We learned that turtles eat fresh fish.

Then came two years at the Walnut Apartments. All the equipment moved, and the turtles' program remained unchanged. Doing what they always did -- nothing.

Then the move to Diastole, and now a 50-gallon aquarium and liver daily (if the owner remembered). Great, monstrous turtles, 12 inches across.

In December 1982 either Molly or Tommy died. We could never tell them apart. It was winter, the ground was frozen, so decent burial was impossible. We put him or her in the freezer to await spring. Spring came, in fact it came three times before I remembered my duty. In the spring of 1985, Molly/Tommy was buried beneath the redbud tree in the back garden.

The remaining turtle, Molly/Tommy, lived on, and on, and on. A visit to see the turtle became a standard part of a visit to Diastole. Hundreds came to see him. In his turtley way he did become famous. For all visitors he did his act -- nothing. His sole pleasure was an enthusiasm for raw liver. He learned to know the time of feeding and maintained a vigil at the feeding corner. Once a month he was taken to the sink and the algae scrubbed off.

Eighteen years passed since McCrory's. His owner got older. The turtle book said that turtles can live 100 years. What to do? How do you provide for his old age?

In a moment of sheer light, the thought came about Hawaii. Daughter Lark lives there. She likes pets. She helped buy Molly/Tommy originally. She was the rightful owner.

One must be clever about such generosity. Suppose she said she didn't want her 18-year-old turtle? Suppose her husband said the same? How do you get a 10-pound turtle to Hawaii?

The answer was quite simple. You say nothing. You give no hint. By stealth you get him there, put him in their hands, and quickly leave. Rapidly.

Molly/Tommy flew, nestled in my briefcase, Kansas City to San Diego, to Los Angeles, to Honolulu, to Kona, sleeping in the bathtub at night, and other than the airport search, flew away to the golden, peaceful, eternal summer of Hawaii, surely a turtle's Shangri-La.

There he sits, doing nothing, in his new 50-gallon aquarium, looking out on the Pacific. Perhaps the only Mississippi yellow-eared turtle to live so well. I hope someday the children do as much for me.

44. Shaping Wood

Decades ago I was engaged personally in a war with mumps, unaware the rest of the country was involved in a great stock-market crash. I was caught up in the quite logical joy of having a modest illness which kept me out of school.

After the first aches passed, the boredom of a 10-day bed confinement settled in. Mom produced a large bar of Ivory soap, a knife, and a request that I make her a swan. There is considerable merit in carving soap in bed. The chips do not have the scratchiness of wood. In fact, they go quite nicely along with the sheets into the laundry. No sandpaper is needed, and a smooth finish needs but a wetting of the finger.

After the swan and recovery, I graduated to pine and whittling. In my twenties, I began self-instructing myself into the full world of sculpturing out of a block of hard wood: the harder, the better.

The pleasure comes from finding the block of wood, for the wood determines the final result. I don't believe I have ever had a subject in my mind and then sought the piece of wood. The shape of the original chunk of wood, whether it is flat, round, spare, has branches, knots, rot, crotch, and the flow of the grain, becomes the challenge. The task becomes one of what can be brought out of the wood, remembering the piece of raw wood when you are doodling, sketching, or awake at night, and gaining an image of what can be hammered out of the wood. I say "hammered" because I want to convey the hard work involved.

The sheer physical labor involved in reducing a log with bark on it down to a satin-smooth-something is not only vastly more effort than one anticipates, but it is also a very good reason why one's productivity results in but a few dozen lifetime examples. The wood sculptor ends up with a single finished product. There are no mass-production copies, for the end product is not only the figure -- female, male, animal, bird, etc. -- but it is the grain of the wood and the smooth, warm, tactile satisfaction from its touch. To duplicate all of the qualities of the original in mass production is not reachable, for one would need the same flaws and sweep of the grain, something unlikely to happen. The touch of a finger to the metal or plastic copy, the missing warmth, would tell you it is not wood.

Carving into wood, like carving into stone, can be deliberately done. By deliberately, I mean planned. One could have a certain head or figure already shaped in clay and then buy a solid block of wood or marble and carve, cut, chisel, and finally bring out the exact image sought. To tell the whole truth, my skills do not include this ability. "Likeness capturing" talent is very much missing in my makeup. I probably compensate for this inability by claiming there is greater pleasure, indeed greater challenge, in bringing out of the wood some interpretation that is dictated by the wood itself. This claim at least gives me a place to hide. The things I have found in wood reflect this limitation set by the nature of the wood itself, and the limits of my own craftsmanship.

From a small limb of orange wood, I carved a male figure, one arm held high, the other cut off at a mid-point by a flaw in the original branch. It made no sense, but that is what the wood let me do. I can only shrug when someone asks, "Why did you leave off the arm?"

Only once did I start out with the head of a person as a plan and felt apprehension as the features were developed. Each wood chip removed is a commitment. There is no going back to fill in lip or nose. There is exquisite pain in trying to create a likeness. The silence as friends study the finished effort is all the answer needed to make one forsake real-life sculpturing.

What kind of wood gives pleasure? Orange, lemon, and grapefruit are extremely hard, fine-grained, and take a lovely finish; however, their wood is white, almost colorless, without character, and lifeless. Lignum vitae is superbly hard, with interesting shades of blue and green when freshly carved. However, with aging, the wood darkens into an almost black-green, and the sculptured piece loses its shading and depths. Lignum vitae, like cocobolo wood, is simply too hard. I never believed wood could be too hard, but after breaking off the cutting edge of a steel chisel simply striking the wood, I now settle for a happy medium. Cherry, walnut, and mahogany take a superb finish, have good color, and the grain gives interest and dimension to the finished piece. They are hard, but not hostile.

In practice, a suitable piece of wood is surprisingly difficult to find. A large, uncracked, unsplit chunk of hard wood is a rare find; between lumber mill and fireplace there is little left. To attempt too large a piece is an invitation to heartbreak -- the bulkier the piece, the more inevitable the cracking. Drying, shrinking, splitting are all painful, and the well-heated American home does a splendid job.

Each piece you do has a personality, a story. No one else ever quite knows the story. What you were doing, where you were when you found the raw wood, the thoughts you had as all alone you chiseled, pounded, carved, cut away the unneeded wood. The changing of plan as a flaw, a problem, a twist in the wood came forth. The small errors made and the attempts at rectification; the major error made and the desperate attempt to salvage something worthwhile; the heartbreaking changes of the piece as drying and cracking occur.

Then after the crash and collisions of the carving of the piece, the silence and carefulness of the filing, the sanding, the waxing, and bringing it to a high gloss. The satisfaction in sitting back, cocking your head, adjusting the light, and seeing the whole finished piece. The pure pleasure in telling yourself that it is well done, that there is no part of it you were careless about. The satisfaction that the thing can be looked at from every angle, in all quantums of light. In being able to whisper to yourself, "I am satisfied; it is right."

The similarity between these paragraphs and the life of a teacher, or a parent, or physician and their career is intentional.

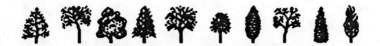

45. Roots, Kansas, and Lea Grey

There is a well-known lumberyard in Kansas City that caters to woodworkers, the kind of men who make beautiful cabinets and chairs. I went there one day on the off-chance that among their woods might be a piece suitable for carving. The clerk was so uninterested and so irritating that I resolved never to return. Near the cash register, I saw a stack of calling cards giving the name of the manager. I handed the alienating clerk one of the cards and said I wanted to speak to the manager. After a snarl or two, he produced him. This man was so cheerful looking, so pleasant, so cordial, that I shifted gears and, without advance clever thinking, I came out with the announcement that I was seeking a major piece of wood, something suitable for formidable sculpting.

I didn't exactly say so, but probably suggested by my demeanor that I knew what I was talking about. Somehow I perhaps expanded the truth about my professionalism. He became enthusiastic but then apologized and said they had nothing of the nature I was seeking. I got all the way out to my car, and there he caught up with me and said he had just remembered three big, ugly pieces of mahogany that had lain in the storeroom for years and maybe I could do something with them. It would be a relief to get rid of them. He would sell the lot for $25. The pieces were huge, ugly, with cracks and rot; they had not been cut on the square. They were ungainly rejects.

As I dug into the crack and rot on the first piece, it became an alarming fault carrying deep into the wood until I was left with an upper and lower chunk of wood connected by a shrunken, central column. I turned the odd-looking thing, stood it one way and another, and finally decided I would make a tree -- a bonsai -- a wooden bonsai.

As I worked away, this plan became more and more vapid to me. Why spend so much effort making something one can achieve by the simple act of going to a nursery? Why do something with wood and knife that nature does better? This kind of reasoning has always been a part of my illogical logic when it comes to wood sculpturing. Why spend the large requirement of effort making a realistic, true-to-life anything? Let the end result be something fully imagined, something not made by man or nature. Call it creative if you are willing. However, realism is not my intent when doodling or chiseling. Nor my ability.

I dropped the idea of a bonsai and began visualizing a tree as a symbol of family. In the months preceding this piece, I had been working on a genealogy about my family. The heritage theme came naturally, with the strong central trunk supported by roots of varying size and length. The top for limbs, too, were all different in length and strength. The roots would be the origins; the trunk the family; the branching limbs the offspring. I had the oak tree in mind as I attempted to interpret its gnarling and twisting, the bends and turns of its branches suggesting the angles and turns of each lifetime.

As I began shaping the final piece and stood back and squinted at it, I saw suddenly that it all had a central theme. A powerful, aged figure -- the trunk -- seemed to support all this on his broad shoulders, and his torso flowed down, out into the roots. This seemed all too clever, and it was not until my daughter Lea Grey saw it and immediately exclaimed, "But Pop, it's not only a tree, there is an old strong man in it, too!" that I was satisfied.

The second piece not only had several cracks,

but one end of it had been cut into a very oblique, slanted angle, which was a fact to be reckoned with.

For many years I had carried an affection for the State of Kansas. The quality of the people in the face of the extremes of climate was an image I carried with me. About 1952 I built a house out in the country south of Kansas City, a home of very modern design with large banks of glass facing south, and eaves projecting out over them. For eight years we lived there. The isolation of the house, its particular shape with its southern angling exposure and scooping eaves, had left in my memory the absolutely unremitting south wind, wind that began some place out in New Mexico, never ceasing, never easing, always leaning on the house.

The wind was such a persistent part of the experience of Kansas life that the Indian tribe of the region had been called the *Kansa*, meaning south wind or people of the south wind. The constancy of the wind, the moaning and humming of the house, the way the wind would drive rain in through the edging of the windows and lift the very texture of the roof to find a hole -- the dust and pollen brought in the summer and fall -- all of these things made the south wind a very real presence. In fact, when Lea Grey was born, it seemed logical to name her Kansas, just out of respect for the character of the region. We finally chose Lea Grey, but as her personality developed, I often regret that she was not Kansas. This thought remained so strong that she and I have acquired the custom of referring to her as The Big Wind. My letters to her often begin with the salutation: Dear Big Wind.

The image I have carried -- the allegory -- of South Wind, has been that of a powerful, feminine figure, with features that were aloof, haughty, passionate. A lovely woman, young, but not too young, intelligent, possessed within, and with great bold waves of hair lifted in the wind. The size of the piece did not allow for a bosom, but if it had, this would have been generous, penetrating.

When Kansas was done, it was a she, the exact she I had sought. From the misshapen, abandoned piece of mahogany, there was Kansas.

These two pieces, *Roots* and *Kansas*, were satisfying to sculpt. The third piece of wood became *The Phoenix* --- but that is another story.

46. Rubaiyatiana

I don't know when I first heard the line, "The moving finger writes, and having writ, moves on ... ", but it must have been a part of things my father said, for it seems I have always been aware of that sentiment. "A loaf of bread, a jug of wine ... " was almost a colloquial expression, and I am referring to Terre Haute, Indiana, where very little poetry was recited.

Not in our home, and not at Purdue or Indiana University do I recall seeing, reading, or discussing the *Rubaiyat*. This was not because it was a suppressed or banned book. My generation was unaware of the alleged raciness, the threat to religion, sobriety, family, and home which had delighted youth in the 1890s. It was not until I began collecting the volumes that I learned of its reputation in the Gay Nineties and the considerable yuppie cult of that time which had grown up around its wine-women-and-song message. A pre-yuppie event, I know, but of course each generation has its yuppies.

My formal introduction was in Tokyo, Japan in the fall of 1946. I was responsible as a young medical officer in the 42nd General Hospital for the cardiology service, and for a 40-bed internal medicine ward reserved for officers. This bit of military elitism made for a stimulating practice, for the designation "officer" included the interesting laymen who were coming to Tokyo to participate in the efforts by General MacArthur to democratize Japan. Forty beds was a heavy load, but the variety of medical problems and personalities made it exciting.

I was called to The Grand Hotel, the superb Frank Lloyd Wright creation, to see a guest who was unable to leave his room. The guest was a senior military physician who had just arrived in Japan with the challenging assignment to be consultant in medicine to the Far East Command. His was certainly an impressive title, for the Far East Command included not only all of Japan, but Korea, parts of China, Okinawa, and Saipan.

The guest proved to be quite sick with fever, chills, and cough. I moved him to my service at the General Hospital, and that was the beginning of a valued friendship. His name was Charles Kettig Berle, his rank, colonel. He was a very senior man, already 65, with 30 years of service. He should not have been given this assignment, but with the war just ending and all experienced physicians scrambling to get out, the army medical corps had held him back from retirement and given him this unneeded burden.

It is peripheral to my theme about the *Rubaiyat*, but I insert that his age and precarious health led to a very exciting year for me. As he tried to carry the burden of his consultancy, which required frequent flights varying from such exciting places as Shanghai to Seoul to Sappora, he began to turn to me and designate me to go as his representative. He kept a firm hold on my decision-making, but the combination of being able to go out and see the problem, see if hospitalization was required in a general hospital, send the patient to my own service in Tokyo, made this a medical experience filled with drama, excitement, challenge, and education.

As he recovered from his pneumonia -- yes, we had penicillin even in that ancient time -- we began an evening ritual that we held to for the remainder of his time in the hospital. I simply wrote an order in his chart for a pitcher of martinis to be delivered each day to his room 30 minutes before dinner. As I finished my afternoon rounds, I slipped into his room and we had our daily "consultation." Col. Berle's physician counterpart, assigned to the Russian delegation, had learned of his illness and sent him a grand supply of caviar. Military duty can have its moments.

On the evening before he was to be discharged, he said he had a gift for me, but first I had to hear the story behind it. Col. Berle had a mellow, resonant voice, had lived long and interestingly, and with his recovery from pneumonia -- and perhaps with the help of my evening medication -- proved to be a charming, witty man and storyteller.

He placed a book on his lap, and said the story began during the First World War during his internship at Louisville General Hospital. A beautiful young girl of 19 was admitted, and he was her physician. An unexplained fever was her problem, and the admission extended for weeks and finally months as she improved but then would have devastating relapses. The young doctor and the lovely girl became friends, good friends, and Col. Berle said, "She was the most perfect person I ever knew."

He became aware that there were never visitors and there were never flowers or letters. The only possession she seemed to have was a book which she read often, and then would tuck back in the drawer of her bedside table. Young Berle finally asked about it and learned that it was the *Rubaiyat of Omar Khayyam.*

The custom grew for him to drop by her bed in the evenings and she would read quatrains to him, each of the young people discussing what the words were saying. The illness was progressive, and it became apparent that she was suffering from subacute bacterial endocarditis, then an absolutely fatal disease. Their sentiment towards each other became one of utter trust and understanding. She never left the hospital, and as the end came, she told him her brief life story. She was raised in an orphanage, had fled, became a prostitute. Her fatal infection was due to a crude abortion. The *Rubaiyat* she had brought from the orphanage was, in the complete sense, her only possession, and now, as she knew her fate, she was giving it to him.

This was a longer story as told by the colonel, and he then leaned back and began reading it, quatrain by quatrain, with a warmth and skill of cadence. Finally, he paused and then handed me the book and said it was mine. He had no children, and he sensed the time had come to pass it on.

Thus it is clear that my formal introduction was exactly the kind of instruction one should have to a writing as emotional and evocative as the *Rubaiyat*. The initial gift launched me on a project that has served me very well. I do enjoy Edward FitzGerald's words, and often have used them or paraphrased them. The phrases are lovely, but I have never found it worth being used as a philosophy or substitute for a religion as so many others have done. The thing itself, the beauty of the words, the beauty of the art the words have provoked, these have been sufficient use of the *Rubaiyat* for me. However, almost more than the sentiment enjoyed from its words, the *Rubaiyat* has been a useful stimulus to give me a bibliophilic interest as a collector.

The hunt for editions I do not have has led me into second-hand bookstores all over the world. Wherever I traveled as a speaker or when attending a medical meeting, I had a delightful reason to slip off to the local bookstore. Old bookstores, the collections in them, the kind of people one finds there, the correspondents one finds, these have been a rare satisfaction. As my collection grew and friends became aware of it, gift Rubaiyats added to my pleasure.

Then came the years when I would get on the trail of a collection and begin the fun of competing, bidding, bargaining, and finally, getting. Visits to bookstores in London, Edinburgh, Dublin had a purpose. I learned of two Omar Khayyam dinner clubs, one in London, one in Boston, whose yearly meetings were a highlight of good food, good wine, and Omar verse. The dinners continued for decades, and each featured an artwork menu, with the art heralding some single verse from the quatrains. Seeking, finding, getting each of these menus epitomizes the collector's fun.

A Mardi Gras in New Orleans was rumored to have been entirely dedicated to the *Rubaiyat*, with each float a quatrain theme and all of the nobles in Arabic dress. Finding the special edition of the *New Orleans Picayune* newspaper, telling of that Mardi Gras in full color, finding it and possessing it. That is satisfaction. Learning that a special *Rubaiyat* had been printed to honor those lost at Pearl Harbor, to not only find it, but to get a lead on the woman living in Honolulu who was involved in its production, only then to learn she had recently died, and that her very substantial collection was in Vermont, to carry out the chase and get it.

To learn that an Egyptian tobacco had been given the name Omar, and that the advertisements used to promote this new cigarette had original artwork based on *Rubaiyat* themes. To learn these ads had been in magazines about 1910, to find them, and to get them in the collection. To hear that a marvelous rabelaisian hand-painted, hand-illuminated, hand-bound leather copy of the *Rubaiyat* existed, and then to confirm that it existed in but a single copy. And get it. To learn an entire *Rubaiyat* opera, from stage play, to costume, to a symphonic orchestration had been done in England, but not to know when or where, and to find not only the program for the performance, but also a handbill for the event, and then to obtain a copy of the symphonic orchestration; to find the smallest edition ever made and get it, but also the microscope needed to read it -- those are the pleasures of book collecting.

Where does such a hobby lead one? With the *Rubaiyat,* I have come to the point which is both satisfying and defeating. Among the thousands of *Rubaiyatiana* in my home, I have managed to acquire a reasonable amount of what is available. Col. Berle's gift is item one in my collection, and it would be a moment of joy to have him see what he set in motion.

Now I have come to the hard part. The hard part being the key items I do not have. The first edition of FitzGerald's translation, the original, is the prime example. It could be obtained, I know it, brokers offer it. However, now we move into that level of commitment which begins to separate a hobby from a business. For me to go ahead and, as the book people say, strengthen my collection, I now need to move into making very large financial commitments. Adding items to my collection has slowed in the last five years, and, for me, this is just about as far as I intend to chase the elegant Tentmaker.

The most handsome edition ever fabricated, in peacock leather and with a handsome peacock on the cover, with each colorful facet of the peacock's plumage set in jewels, is said to have been lost on the Titanic. The thought of having that in one's collection does bring a sparkle to one's eye, and -- who knows?

VI. INTERESTS ABROAD

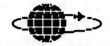

47. Xigatse Stress Test

Cardiologists have many devices for testing the fitness of the heart. Early, there was the two-step exercise test; this gradually evolved and now there are vigorous treadmill stressings to find the outer limits of one's pump. As an advance in this field, I want to offer for scientific study the Xigatse Stress Test.

Xigatse (pronounced ShiGOTsa) is the second-largest city of Tibet, and the monastery there is the home base of the Panchen Lama. The Panchen Lama is the head of the Buddhist faith in Tibet, the head Buddhist-in-residence while the Dalai Lama takes refuge in India. Presently they are seeking a reincarnation of the Panchen; the post is empty.

I arrived in Xigatse on the evening of a three-day religious holiday, an occasion to honor Buddha. This holiday had been suppressed for some 30 years, and the renaissance of the occasion was a huge event. Thirty-thousand pilgrims poured into Xigatse -- "poured in" is an inappropriate expression, for these pilgrims were Tibetans who had trudged in over mountain passes, and some had been on their way for six months.

It was a huge crowd, a quiet crowd, travel-tattered and unbelievably soiled. Just plain dirty. Tibetans are good-looking people, and in their dress, even filthy, are still rather dashing. Men and women, no matter how weathered, have bright splashes of coral and turquoise necklaces and earrings, with a dagger at their belt, making them picturesque, picaresque, and somewhat intimidating to the foreign traveler.

I asked the local guides if our group could go to the monastery and watch the ceremonies. There is where my story gets interesting. I evidently didn't make clear the point "watch the ceremonies," for bright and early the next morning we were herded to the monastery and put down in the midst of this pilgrim mass. Instantly we were swept up into the penultimate act of the pilgrimage, a stress-test for the faithful. This fact was not clear to me in the first 20 minutes, as I thought we were all moving forward to the main temple.

It was not until this stream of mankind swept by the temple and started up the mountain behind it that it dawned on me, dawned on me as a considerable shock, that the local Tibetan guides, perhaps through a malignant sense of humor, had sent these "long-nosed foreign devils" off to participate in and complete the final penance of the pilgrimage.

This event, an ordeal to prove one's devoutness, is done in single file over a long, rocky trail on the mountainside up and behind the monastery. The route is up, over, and around boulders, across loose rock, along ledges, and is done at a great, urgent pace. The Tibetans chant a low prayer, steadily repeating *om mani padme hum, om mani padme hum*, and slip their prayer beads through their fingers as they are hurried along by monks with staves and whips -- yes, whips. Penance includes punishment.

For the Tibetan in his mountain shoes, just in from his vigorous trek to get there, fired up with religious fervor, it was apparent that this was a great moment. I felt keenly my misplacement as an interloper, but also for my group in their casual tourist clothes, their alligator-labeled shirts, their bundles of cameras dangling from their necks. For us, it became not a pilgrimage, but a question of survival. Only the very senior member of our group had the good sense to sit down on a rock and just wait.

The rest of us, typical tourists, thought surely

this path was taking us to see something spectacular. I was up at the head of the group, and we were spread out over a mountainside on this torture trail and I could not get word back to them that there was nothing up ahead to see but more up.

At 13,000 feet, in penetrating bright sun, we rushed up, up, up, across, across, down, down with earnest monks pressing us on as fast as we could move. All of us were slipping, scrambling, stumbling in an effort to keep up, hang on to our cameras, our hats, our dignity, our very lives. I had no breath to spare for the constant Bhuddist chant: *om mani padme hum*.

Upon completing this mountain circle, one has gained some extra step towards rebirth, but for our group, survival was the reward. One of our group, a rather portly man said, "Dammit, Grey, I am paying a fortune for this experience. Back home, I'm afraid to have a Bruce Stress Test, and here, two miles high, you run me around like a mountain goat."

For those who have a chronic anxiety about the adequacy of their cardiovascular systems, I am offering my services as both physician and travel agent to arrange for them to have this ultimate stress test. Upon passing the test, one can have superb confidence in the adequacy of their heart. If one fails the test, there is a very thorough Tibetan burial ceremony utilizing buzzards that is included in the tour package.

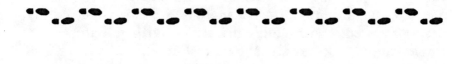

48. The Joy of the Journey

I need to report a recent excursion I made from the Hill. From my home on Hospital Hill, I went to some much higher hills, namely the Himalayas. It gives me obvious pleasure to report I got back in good health. No pulmonary edema, no angina. Everything worked, nothing fell off. We were above 13,000 feet for several days, and at about 16,000 feet for several hours. One moves slowly and thoughtfully at that altitude; from there on up, even the healthiest can have pulmonary edema.

Our group traveled across Tibet, northeast to southwest, for some 600 miles, from Lhasa to the Nepal border, down to Katmandu. I felt it was a quite heroic adventure. I was brought down to size, deflated, by two events, however. The first of these leveling events was the fact that in my party was an 88-year-old woman doctor who had absolutely no difficulty with altitude, corrugated roads, clouds of dust, unflushable toilets. In fact, for two days no toilets of any sort, just open high plateau. That grand old gal sailed along, cheerfully, enthusiastically, healthfully. I had to act healthy even if I felt miserable, just to keep up with her. She made 88 seem young.

The other deflating experience, reminding me that I was not Marco Polo or Neil Armstrong, but simply an American tourist in a Japanese bus, cosseted by guides, occurred about 200 miles west of Xigatse, on the road to Zhangmu. This is an empty, desolate area, with one primitive village along the whole route. It is all above tree-line, with no shade, just intense, bright sun and penetrating wind, an occasional herd of yak, and a thin scatter, very thin, of herdsmen.

I was trying to ease my pounded bottom, clear my nostrils of dust, my throat of grit, and marvel at our act of heroism in making this crossing, when to my amazement, we came upon a man, a Caucasian, on his bicycle, all alone, a tent and sleeping bag on the back of his bike. He had already ridden from Kathmandu to Lhasa, seen the sights, and was now peddling his way back over this tortuous road to Kathmandu.

My emotions were a mix of envy and sympathy. To be 21, to have that adventure, to have the imagination to do it, made it difficult to suppress a surge of jealousy and a depression in knowing the time for my doing it was past.

My envy was tempered a bit from noting the almost blank expression about his face and eyes. He obviously was going to succeed, for when we met him he was two-thirds done with the trip. However, his gauntness, desiccation, and blunted affect left no doubt that he was scraping the bottom of his physical and emotional reserves. He still had to reach the last, highest pass, at 16,200 feet when we saw him, but from that point to Katmandu, it is a downhill rollercoaster.

The last day of his journey would need no peddling, but I hoped he had effective handbrakes. The descent from the Everest plateau to the Nepal border is one of the great roadway experiences of the world. The Amalfi Drive is a toy in comparison.

His fatigue will go, the glow will come back to his eyes, and the rest of his life he can remember the joy of this journey and the satisfaction of using the power of his body. If I could give everyone the perfect graduation gift, I would have them all on bicycles making the round-trip from Kathmandu to Lhasa.

49. Forty-three Hours in Moscow

Travel light, travel quick. Good rules. Avoid the heavy luggage and stay in motion.

Come with me on a trip to Moscow: Land there at 10:30 a.m. on Monday, leave at 5:30 a.m. on Wednesday. Elapsed ground time: 43 hours.

Leave Kansas City on Sunday; back in your own bed on Wednesday night.

That takes care of "travel quick." What about "travel light?" Simple. Check your bag in at Kansas City airport, see it again 42 days later. Lost luggage guarantees light travel. Also guarantees wearing same shirt for four days.

One dividend of such travel is an absence of jet lag; you're back home before your body has had time to lag.

Forty-three hours in Moscow were divided into 14 hours of sleeping, four hours of eating, two hours of hunting lost luggage, two hours of drinking beer, two hours of scrambling for a ticket home, two hours of conference, two hours of coming and going from the airport, and 15 hours of sightseeing.

This may seem to be a record for futile travel, but the single two-hour conference was completely effective. All items on the agenda were settled. The trip was a success. If I had stayed longer, I would have been a burden to my hosts. And my shirt would have become a burden to all.

Forty-three hours of observation of a vast foreign city may seem as unproductive as doing a museum on a galloping horse. However, what you see, you see. Here are synoptic extractions:

Moscow is so very European. You could believe you were in Vienna, Budapest, even Paris. Boulevards, esplanades, gardens, monuments, public buildings, statues, all the splendor of a national capital. One reads of the lack of color, but this seemed no more absent than in other northern European cities. Although October, the flowers were impressive, and even tuberous begonias were in bloom.

Trams, trolleys, taxis, trucks, private cars, and big-city traffic. The subway a handsome, people-packed world, with shops, newsstands, flower stalls, and crowds moving at a bustling pace, intent, purposeful.

The weather was topcoat pleasant. The birch trees were golden, and the sidewalks were as peopled as the subway. Family groups, often three generations; dating couples acting like dating couples; sidewalk cafes still busy although late in the season; an obvious teen-age culture in international dress, with jeans, jogging shoes, colorful sweatshirts. An occasional punk haircut.

Younger women very much using eye shadow and mascara. Surprising popularity of an orange-red henna hair rinse among women of all ages. Equally surprising popularity of silver and gold-threaded pantyhose, the weight of the metallic thread making the hose sag at the ankles. One nice-looking man in his thirties, dumb-drunk on his knees. Robed, orthodox priests -- handsome, bearded men.

Of course, the improbable architecture and exuberant color of the old churches, standing out in the gray city like unrelated movie sets.

The phenomenon that is The Gum, in its own way a wonder of the world: a giant series, sequence, and strategy of merchandising. Three immense arcades, glass-roofed fountains -- surely the grandparent of all shopping malls. Three separate buildings, each three stories high, each with tiers of shops with a central atrium, all joined at a center, all distinct in pastel coloring, a blue, a green, a beige arcade.

Much more merchandise than I had expected -- a galaxy of shops, each with a special purpose: shoes, hats, gloves, kitchenware, pastries, clocks, eyeglasses, luggage, knives, cameras, shirts, blankets. Imagine two miles of shops arranged in tiers, packed with people and frequent queues.

All this in a society of rationing and shortages. As a piece of nineteenth-century architecture, it is its own treasure.

The beer cellars looking like Munich or Amsterdam. Iced steins of draft beer, Heinekens. Dozens of earnest conversations, obviously where you bring a date and where the bachelors hang out. A no-nonsense frowning matron keeping control. The nearby restaurant bringing in a dance band after 9 o'clock, and a quite stylish crowd in for later dinner and cheek-to-cheek 1930s dancing.

A table set up on the sidewalk in front of the hotel and the bakery department practicing a little private endeavor, selling cakes, and a 30-person queue quickly forming.

The interior of the churches, some a museum, some active, heaped with the red and gold splendor of icons. My university escort a resource of historical information -- a sweep of knowledge blending in Peter the Great, Ivan the Terrible, Catherine the Great, Alexander, Nicholas -- and my quiet personal resolve to review Russian history.

The range of the political geography told in the impressive number of Asians, the city so European, but the people both European and Asian. A heterogeneity just as in the United States, but with the absence of the African-American.

The hockey arena advertising the coming of a famed Soviet rock band.

The determination of Moscow University to pay an honorarium and the bureaucracy set in motion: The check authorized in a specific room in a specific building. The honorarium paid by check in a certain building in a certain room up long stairs. The requirement that the check be cashed in a designated building in a designated way, and all three points of action separated by considerable distances. Then, with rubles in hand, learning they could not be taken from the country, could not be converted into dollars, could not be used to pay my hotel bill, and finally, putting them away as a souvenir.

The Kremlin, Red Square, St. Basil's Cathedral, all as real, impressive, and characteristic of Moscow as the Forbidden City and the Temple of Heaven are of Beijing; as the Lincoln, the Washington, and the Jefferson memorials are of Washington.

And of course, the necessary moment of ordering caviar with vodka and its arrival at the table: a crystal service of caviar on ice, small plates of dry toast, chopped egg and onion, and a flagon of vodka plunged into a bed of ice.

All this in 43 hours. What one could do in a week ...

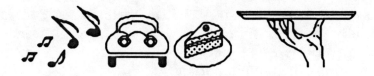

50. Basic Hopes and Fears

Some will remember the days of World War II, Korea, and Vietnam, when a form of nomenclature grew up, a nomenclature in which we identified letters by words: A-Able, B-Baker, C-Charlie, and so on became an absolute of communication. As a biased American, I thought that this was world standard.

There is a new era we are entering, the era of the Pacific Basin. Economic dominance is moving to the East, and many reading this are destined to live in the age of Pacific Basin dominance.

This was brought home to me in a minuscule manner when I stepped up to the counter of Singapore Airlines in Singapore. I wanted to confirm my ticket, my name was Dimond. The pert, quite attractive Chinese girl picked up the phone and then began to identify the spelling of my name to the listener. No D-Dog, but quite rapidly; D-Djakarta, I-Indonesia, M-Malaysia, O-Osaka, N-Nagasaki, D-Djakarta. It was all so logical, so correct, so unexpected, so much a reminder of what a large world there is beyond ABLEBAKERCHARLIE.

I grew up in a society that felt naturally akin to Europe. Our cultural roots, religious ties, our very genes made us think the United States and Europe -- especially western Europe -- were the "world," and the other parts were exotic, or wishing-to-be-like-us, or, quite often, just unimportant.

From the earliest days of my training in cardiology, I began learning there were other interpretations of this world. My teachers were not all physicians, but three very different personalities with different routes through life, who all arrived at quite similar beliefs about the world, the world's peoples, and how to have a stabilized international social system. The three men were Paul Dudley White, cardiologist; Grenville Clark, lawyer; and Edgar Snow, journalist.

These job descriptions are incomplete, for each man was more than the label I just used. They were "complete" men. I use this word to mean that each had reached the level of genuine understanding and tolerance which let them be comfortable within themselves and fully able to accept all variations of race, belief, and politics.

They were Americans, but they were men of the world. Not a *bon vivant* world, but three men comfortable with concepts of equality, rationality, and a global harmony. They were not naive, not in the least; they were not lost in a dream of perfecting mankind. They were not even unbiased or unprejudiced. However, they had sufficient wisdom to know there is always another side to a story, and that you (as one said to me), "... can get from here to there by giving a little, helping a little, accepting a little -- and if you are right, the other fellow will begin to do it your way. If you are wrong, then think it over, perhaps you can learn something."

The three men all realized the *realpolitik* facts that there would be no prospect of world harmony unless the vast Chinese civilization was brought into social networks of law, banking, corporations, insurance, shipping, import-export, air and rail, schooling, professional standards. Not issues regulating how a people worship or choose their government, but international manners and rules of propriety.

In 1971, on the very day the new Medical School in Kansas City opened, I entered China, invited by Zhou Enlai, directly through the endorsement of American journalist Edgar Snow. I invited Dr. White to go with me, and I went to Snow's home in Switzerland to get my briefing. We could not include Grenville Clark, for he had died in 1967, but his daughter did go.

Not because of our visit to China has the great burst of Sino-American friendship occurred, but we were able to be at least visible evidence that it was possible to pass through the Bamboo Curtain, come home, and tell those who trusted us that there were indeed people of good faith there, as here.

Ed Snow died the week President Nixon landed in Shanghai. Paul White died in 1976, but the deaths of Clark, Snow, and White were of little consequence, as the momentum of U.S.-China communication poured forth. They would have endorsed my use of the term "little consequence", for a part of their completeness was an awareness of the transitory nature of a single life and how it is but a moment on the continuing tide on earth. They were but drops, but they well knew that the course of the river can change when a sufficient volume of water seeks a new path.

The wise person continues to travel, to study, to seek to understand the variations and varieties of humankind, and ultimately to realize how similar are basic hopes and fears -- everywhere. It is that lesson, well-learned, that is the true objective of a liberal education.

51. Why?

Physicians usually take care of people one at a time. It is that one-to-one relationship, the quality of it, that distinguishes the caring physician from the technician. It is the area in which our patients find fault or comfort. Here, I want to talk about a larger practice: the world.

My message is very simple, but to gain your attention, I must complicate it by numbers. I cannot apologize; the numbers are the lesson. I want to talk about numbers of people on earth. Don't tense. I am not taking up the cudgel for birth control. Nor am I slipping in a warning about the potential for famine or pollution.

Let the numbers speak for themselves. The long, long list below is the estimate of the population of each country by 1995. Not a distant date, but one essentially all readers will live to experience. The countries are grouped roughly by continent.

All these countries with all of their people and all of their talent that is living, dying, contributing, warring, procreating, purchasing, and other things of life equal one-billion, two-hundred and forty-seven million, eight-hundred thousand souls.

Reflect on each country's individuality, the talent of their people, their contributions to history, literature, music, art, the wars fought, the iceboxes, television sets, and cars used.

Think of the time and space each of these nations captures in our newspapers and on our television sets.

Think of the diplomatic time, the legislative energy, the commercial endeavors these countries expend. Think, even of the amount of the U.S.

taxpayer's money used.

Read the list slowly, reflecting on the people you have known from each country; think of the importance of both country and individual to the world's personality.

I am often asked why I think it important to devote time and energy to China. The population of China in 1995 will be 1,255,700,000-- one billion, two hundred and fifty-five million, seven-hundred thousand. Yes, China's population is but matched by that of all these countries. Think about it.

CHINA (1995)   1,255,700,000

The population of all these nations (1995) just matches that of China.

Ethiopia	50,000,000
Zimbabwe	12,600,000
Algeria	30,500,000
Egypt	58,900,000
Libya	5,200,000
Sudan	28,700,000
Cuba	11,200,000
Haiti	8,600,000
El Salvador	7,500,000
Nicaragua	4,500,000
Mexico	99,200,000
Argentina	35,100,000
Chile	14,000,000
Bolivia	8,400,000
Columbia	34,900,000
Peru	25,100,000
Canada	28,300,000
Japan	127,700,000
South Korea	46,800,000

Iran	58,700,000
Iraq	21,600,000
Israel	5,000,000
Jordan	5,200,000
Saudi Arabia	16,100,000
Bulgaria	9,600,000
Czechoslovakia	16,300,000
Hungary	10,600,000
Poland	40,200,000
Romania	24,800,000
Denmark	5,100,000
Finland	5,000,000
Ireland	4,000,000
Norway	4,200,000
Sweden	8,100,000
United Kingdom	56,000,000
Greece	10,500,000
Italy	57,900,000
Portugal	10,700,000
Spain	42,000,000
Yugoslavia	24,600,000
Austria	7,500,000
France	56,300,000
Germany	76,800,000
Netherlands	14,900,000
Switzerland	6,000,000
Australia	17,700,000
New Zealand	3,600,000
TOTAL	1,247,800,000

My point needs little editorial comment.

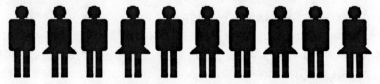

52. What is the Margin of Truth?

We Westerners read of traditional doctors in China -- the herbal, acupuncture doctors. One needs to understand an often forgotten merit of traditional Chinese medicine: it is economical in terms of use of health care providers. There are 700,000 traditional physicians in China now working "in the system," absorbing a vast number of the initial health complaints of 1 billion plus people. This "style" of medical practice is inexpensive; acupuncture and herbs are far removed from the cost range of modern X-rays, laboratory tests, and prescriptions.

All of us, medical professionals and the general public, should have a continuing degree of scorn for the wild claims of acupuncture. However the scientific evidence that the process of acupuncture results in the brain's release of a pain-suppressing chemical comes very close to offering a livable answer. There is a logical, vast overuse of acupuncture in China. It is one means that has helped in the dilemma of how to handle the medical care of a huge population. Even if the procedure is not likely to become a standard in America, one has the challenge posed by the Chinese success with acupuncture anesthesia and the increasing literature defining neurophysiological and neurochemical mechanisms.

American medical literature has not helped by its eagerness to deny any possible neuropharmacological explanations. An example of this occurs in the tone of the heading of an editorial that appeared in the Journal of the American Medical Association. The title? "Acupuncture Anesthesia: Pricking the Balloon." The author presents facts about acupuncture, presents them negatively. Yet in the body of his editorial he finds himself able to write of his own experience in China: "Of the six intrathoracic operations [including one repair of a ventricular septal defect under extra-corporeal circulation] only one [of the patients] was not covered satisfactorily by [acupuncture anesthesia]."

Translated, this means that six humans had their chests opened surgically, including one who had his heart opened, also, and a hole in it repaired. Five of the six required no "anesthetic other than acupuncture." Some balloon! Some pricking! The editorial fails to explain the ability to open the chest in six patients, plus the heart in a sixth, with pain obtunded by wiggling a needle placed three-fourths of an inch deep in the forearm.

The Chinese success in limb replantation, in the salvage of third-degree burns, in the willow-splint treatment of fractures are equally potential fields for us to study.

Scientific analysis of the ingredients of traditional medicine may well be the major benefit to the world. Every day, millions of Americans take trusted medications that have come from folklore knowledge. Digitalis, morphine, quinine, ephedrine, and cascara are examples of the vindication of our ancestral herbal enthusiasts.

The reported results in China about herbal medicine will need very thoughtful appraisal. Enthusiasts may oversell. However, as we enter this Pacific Rim era, one needs a balance: an open mind, a cautious mind.

In September 1971, Paul White and I were exposed to a full barrage of herbs, acupuncture, acupuncture for deafness, and acupuncture anesthesia. We also were the guests in Peking of the medical leadership, men and women with the highest degree of medical and surgical sophistication. By no shadow of wording did they fault the role of acupuncture in, for example, the treatment of deafness. This new relationship between us was precise, well-mannered and cordial, but unremittingly cautious. No negative remarks were made about traditional medicine. The steady phrase was, "It has not all been worked out yet. It is being studied."

In January 1979, I was at a reception in Washington, D. C. given by the Chinese government. This was after the Cultural Revolution, and after the Chinese had announced that they sought world assistance to gain modernization. They stated that the Cultural Revolution cost them 10 years -- a lost generation of talent.

Suddenly, I was gently tugged by the elbow, and standing there was a Chinese physician who had been one of my hosts in Peking in 1971. He said, "I must tell you now that much of what was told you about acupuncture in 1971 was not correct -- in fact, some of it was actually not the truth."

We smiled at each other beneficently, each looking at the other's eyes for seconds. He said, "I know you will understand." I nodded, and he moved quietly across the room.

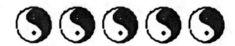

53. Much More Than Herbs and Acupuncture

Several years ago, I wrote a book about China that I titled, *More Than Herbs and Acupuncture*. I was striving to report to an American reading audience that we must not blind ourselves to the tremendous rate of change in China as it makes its drive for industrialization and a return to prime position among the world's premier nations. Don't tuck China away as an exotic land with a great wall, and perhaps some clever ideas in their folklore medicine, but not much else.

The need for such a warning was put in capsule form for me when one of my American friends analyzed the prospects for a vigorous, prosperous new China by saying, "They will never amount to anything. All my life I have heard about the promising potential for China and still all they have are floods, famines, war lords, earthquakes, revolts". The fact that my friend was 60 years old and "all my life", which he used as his time frame, was a somewhat scanty sample of Chinese history, he, nevertheless, probably expressed the sentiment of the majority of Americans.

Many of us find comfort in cataloging, labeling, pigeon-holing China by thinking of it as a mysterious sleepy landscape of buffalo and improbable mountains.

Although the title of my book sought to emphasize that one was misled in understanding today's China if the image carried was one of quaint herbal medicine and acupuncture, readers absolutely ignored the critical word "more" in my title. Instead of serving as a warning that I believed there was immense progress in modern China, and that the drive towards regaining their world status was succeeding, I was immediately identified as an expert on herbs and acupuncture.

Bookstores put the book in the holistic medicine section, and letters and telephone calls poured in. Could I see Aunt Matilda at once? Her arthritis was awful, and she needed acupuncture. Could I send some reindeer horn immediately? Some peony root? Could I speak and give a clinic in Las Vegas on surgery under acupuncture anesthesia?

No matter how vigorously I declared I knew nothing about acupuncture and my only message was to say that China was returning to the world scene, I was extolled as an expert on herbs and acupuncture. When I reflected that I had spent my entire career in attempting a reputation in cardiology and now, without even the pretext of any skill in these odd and inexplicable therapies, I could have had instant public acceptance and prosperity, it was humbling and alienating.

Finally, the confusing and disturbing message registered. The lesson was that a sick person wants help, and the help does not need to be scientific or even "approved." In fact, I painfully learned the appeal of the exotic, the unknown, was in itself a prime factor in the public's enthusiasm. The charm came in part from its *ex cathedra*, outside-the-establishment, nature.

This enthusiasm was not transitory. It continues down to the present, and each trip I make to China with a group has as its high point the visit to an outpatient clinic, where all the members of the travel party, lay people and physicians leap about, oohing, ahhing, cameras flashing, recording for the discussion group back home the wonders of cupping, moxa, acupuncture, and a fragrant, huge pharmacopeia of bear bile, ground pearl, rhinoceros horn, and chrysanthemum leaves.

Someplace in all of these trusted drugs there are undoubtedly some fragments of truth. Adequate real research will find the truth and fit them into a scientific logic. Much will not be verified but scientific opinion will probably not deter the American holistic enthusiast. In China, although it will assuredly be a great, industrialized world-power, one can feel confident that there will continue to be a vast faith and use of traditional medicine.

Is this bad? No, I don't think so. One of the primary ingredients of healing is faith, a trust, an abiding belief. The title of my book was a mistake, but it served to remind me of the healing quality of trust -- and that when one is sick there is no limit to the reaching one will do for help. A physician handicaps and interferes with the human equation who does not leave room for those unknown factors that, perhaps "unscientifically," are based on faith.

It was not the exact meaning I was seeking, but there is something more than herbs and acupuncture.

54. The Return of China

In my adult life, I have been repeatedly in China. The most important thing I have learned is to not draw a conclusion. What one sees is a fact of the moment.

In Medicine we seek to make a diagnosis by taking pieces of tissue, a biopsy. We assume that a small bit of sample is an example of the whole.

My lesson in China is that there is no adequate biopsy. My conclusion is that the only way to understand this world called China is by once or twice a year house calls, a feeling of the pulse and a look at the tongue, appear wise and cheerful, and then go home, keeping your conclusions inside.

Often my visits to China have been in the name of Edgar Snow. Increasingly, and now in a rush, I find that I am the only American in my group who ever knew him. Even in China where he had unique contacts, those who knew him are coming down to a few.

Recently an Associated Press reporter came to see me. He came because he had learned that at my university there was an Edgar Snow Memorial Fund. The reporter, about 30 years old, in complete openness and good faith, asked me who was Ed Snow. Even when in China, where the memory of Snow is maintained by government policy, I am asked very frequently by my young contacts, such as guides, drivers, even young physicians "who was Snow?"

In truth the man is dead, dead more than 20 years, and his message from Paoan and Yenan is history. What he wrote about has happened. His efforts of 60 years ago, all of his writing and reporting about what he learned in his 14 years in China, of course remains. They are history, items for the library and classroom analysis as examples of skilled journalism.

The facts of yesterday are out of date but his basic message remains: to tell the world that it must understand the significance of China. Now, even more, that is the largest international message of our time.

Snow's burden was that the United States did not want to hear that message. It was contrary to public desire, contrary to political purpose. Very few could appreciate that his message was not the Communists, but the return of the Chinese people as one of the world's great nations.

That is the role I have cast for myself. My message through all of the years has been that the ancient Middle Kingdom has healed itself and the rest of the world must factor in this significance. The assault on China, beginning in the 1840s, lasted more than a hundred years. We Americans have scant awareness of the history that preceded ourselves. For several generations, we were brought up on a diet of Boxer Rebellion, gun-boat diplomacy, foreign concessions, a falling empire, war-lords, social disasters, civil wars, cultural revolution. We became victims of our exposure and forgot that for thousands of years there had been a large, stable, and significant Chinese nation.

My own small approach to persuading my peer Americans has been to have a spectrum of them see this for themselves. I have not sought to invest money in this new China but have invested time and energy. I do not even attempt to be a messenger, instead I have taken the route of facilitating the natural harmony between the two people. Chinese and Americans fit each other. Their humor, their robustness, their courtesy fit each other.

I come at this with moral intent as did my

teacher Paul White and my father-in-law, Grenville Clark. My belief is that there can never be world harmony unless vast China is heard and respected.

We Americans convince ourselves that we are what all other countries would like to be, if they were but "free". That may be true or it may not be. When dealing with such a large power as China we need to accept them as they are. Through our example and through full contact, we need to allow two-way communication to carry the message. They will determine their own changes.

There are only two great world powers. One is old China, recovering its prominence after 150 years. The other, a new country, a new people, a new concept -- unheard of when China was last a great power. Now in the 21st century, the job, the need, the hope is that they understand and respect each other.

55. Simmons Fred Slept Here

George Bernard Shaw is credited with saying that the United States and Great Britain are two great nations divided by a common language.

English-English and American-English, the same language when written, become almost foreign when rendered into the spoken word and serve to separate, rather than bind.

Therefore it is not a surprise that communication becomes overwhelmingly difficult if two people try to communicate when one uses the Western alphabet, and the other, Chinese calligraphy characters. Magnifying the inability to exchange is the historical and cultural background upon which each language has grown. An illustration is the story of Fred Simmons.

At dinner one evening, there were two Americans and five Chinese. The menu was Italian. We were having lasagna. Five Chinese, two Americans, and Italian food.

The five Chinese were on a three-week tour of the United States seeking to develop cultural, academic, and commercial ties. Three of the Chinese had a technical college education, one, the leader, had not been schooled, and the fifth man was a graduate of the Foreign Languages Institute. He was the group's interpreter. It was heavy going. The evening seemed endless. The lasagna was good.

One of the salvations of such an evening is the Chinese custom of an early ending to the evening. I began slipping looks at my watch. Then, suddenly, an interesting exchange occurred which made the whole evening priceless.

Because the interpreter was the only guest with

whom I could have a casual word, I found it comfortable to ask him, "What was the range of the curriculum at the Foreign Languages School?" I was interested in learning if their exposure included anything about Western society. They studied the language, obviously, but what did they learn about the people who spoke it?

The interpreter nodded and explained that it was a full, four-year curriculum, which he believed was very similar to a liberal arts degree in our country. Yes, they had studied politics, Western history, social sciences, etc. . . . "For example?" I asked.

He studied for a moment and then, quite brightly, said, "Well, we learned about Simmons Fred!"

I reflected, and thoughtfully suggested he tell me more about it. This gentle urging was taken as a challenge, and he was flustered for a moment, then said, "We learned about his bed!"

The other American and I glanced at each other, shrugged, and I suggested hesitantly, "Perhaps you are talking about the Simmons bed? Perhaps a lecturer talked about the typical American home life and described our soft beds and our Simmons mattresses? They are popular, that is true."

The interpreter was thoroughly confused by this effort of mine, and responded, "No. No! This was a medical bed, a special place for patients!"

Happily, I nodded and said, "Oh, you mean Saunders bed, not Simmons. Yes, years ago, there was a rocking bed used in medicine especially for lung and heart disease. Yes. You mean a Saunders bed!"

This remark, on top of my mattress suggestion, sunk the interpreter, and he struggled to inform me.

"No, not a mattress, and not a rocking bed. The patient rested on it, and the doctor sat by it -- Simmons Fred!"

Then the interpreter threw out one extremely

slender ray of light. He volunteered, "You know, we understood that he was a very famous doctor. He knew all about dreams and childhood, and problems of that sort."

There it was. The clues were in. The answer was obvious. Two great people separated by an uncommon language.

My guest was reaching back into his memory of college courses and had come up with one of the basic units of Western vocabulary. Of course! We all knew Simmons Fred and his bed.

No mattress, no rocking. Simmons Fred, the man who sat by the bed and knew about dreams and childhood problems of that sort? Sigmund Freud! Our Chinese guest had a phonetic recall, words he had not understood in the first place. Simmons Fred was just as logical as Sigmund Freud.

The evening was a great success. I was still smiling after I had shown them to the door. I went back to the untidy table, picked up one of their unemptied glasses, raised it, and said, "Simmons Fred! To your health!"

VII. TYING IT ALL TOGETHER

56. Eternal Verities

One of the problems for a senior physician in essay-writing is gap, age gap. Almost all those who read it are in younger years; the man who writes is, to be gentle, in his fully mature years.

What he writes must walk a shifting line between patronizing, sermonizing, and harmonizing. Nothing can overcome that ultimate resistance when the younger reader rapidly turns away and mutters, "The old fogey is about to tell about the good old days again."

The writer may, even within himself, think that he is still current with the changing scene, "with it," but reality is that decades separate writer and reader. The secret to such a communication dilemma is obvious. One must write about the eternal verities, the basic truths that are fundamental. Their labels may change and their presence may seem to be a new discovery for each generation, but surely they exist.

The young reader is forming her or his opinions, seeing and hearing the issues anew, weighing the rightness, sifting for the truth through one's own maze of bigotry. Part of youths' response to age gap is to reject the answers given by the elders. If this did not happen, each generation would not so happily, thoroughly, energetically repeat the errors of its parents.

One sits with pen in hand, poised, ready, full of well-aged wisdom, eager to find a disciple -- and caution clogs the pen, the paper, the mind. Discretion falters the intent. Enthusiasm sinks beneath the burden. Fire in the soul fails under the weight of prudence.

Old men know what is right. Fortunately, the

young do not. Life still moves forward. A new generation may solve the eternal problems a little more accurately, more reasonably, more gently. Each generation expresses its own genius in its own way. That is the hope that sustains. That is the eternal verity.

57. All Hung Out: Shore-to-Shore

For eighteen years I made a monthly medical audiotape. The audience was always the physician. One month I referred to Dr. Ruth and her sex column. Phone calls and letters came in to tell me that Tape Four was the best tape I had ever made. I enjoyed this sudden burst of listener-enthusiasm and listened to the tape to see what I had done to deserve accolade. I had done nothing different -- the tape was popular because of my kibitzing of Dr. Ruth's sex column. My good listeners (and their spouses) simply enjoyed my foray into saltier subjects.

This set me to thinking, reflecting on other observations that one makes in a medical lifetime in the United States. I thought of the most widely read journalist, and of course it is Ann Landers. Her style is to let the public ventilate itself, usually on questions of sex, although not always, and then she constructs an answer which is a saucy mix of wit, liberalism, and -- almost always -- ends by telling the writers that they should "get counseling."

Think about life in this country. We are a nation engaged in group therapy. Not only are the most successful columnists a part of this group effort, but when one browses through a book store, the shelves are loaded with let-it-all-hang-out authors who essentially do a 180-page Ann Landers column and put it in hardback. The authors almost always describe some major problem that brought them to the brink: alcoholism, drugs, being abused, being the abuser, inadequacy of, or too much of, or an odd kind of sex life, or having misused the public trust and, thereafter, being born again. It often relates to being born inadequate, unable to function successfully in school, in work, in interpersonal relationships, in, yes, sex -- and then the upbeat conclusion, usually with a simplistic explanation, explaining how some particular event brought about this phenomenal recovery.

Sometimes it is a movie actress who finds all necessary answers through a guru who escorts her through her several reincarnations, or a politician who, during a prison term, finds the Bible has all the answers, or a daughter who, through the act of writing the book, succeeds in placing on a parent the full explanation for the child's complete inadequacy. Strange, isn't it, that practically none of these books is written by parents explaining what an awful experience it had been to be the father or mother of some inadequate child?

The public evidently loves this flood of books telling one how to use extrasensory perception, or how to feel okay 'cause you are okay, or how to find complete mental and physical health through some odd version of science such as colonic irrigation, acupressure, breathing exercises, foot massage, aroma therapy, and/or organic farming.

When you turn to television talk shows and soap operas, it is all the same thing -- group therapy, simply put into technicolored acting, often with tears brought into the performance -- and prayer.

If you analyze us, you will see that we are, sea-to-sea, up to our chins in group therapy. The drama on television or stage is simply putting Ann Landers into images. Our whole world is one vast effort of feeling, purging our inner emotions in public; we are one shore-to-shore arena of let-it-all-hang-out. We seem to have a fear of having one's own thoughts, keeping one's privacy, resolving life's pressures through one's own efforts.

The columnists, the books, the talk shows, the movies -- all cry out that you must be careful and not keep anything within yourself, that such is harmful that you have a duty to your sanity to ventilate, to throw your own two-bits into the national dirty wash, take advantage of the national group therapy and tell everyone about your private problems.

I suppose I should look for the bright side of all this and reflect on how much money it would cost if all of this inadequacy had to find its care on the psychoanalytical couch. All of this self-help must wreck the appointment book of the Freudian therapists, or perhaps I am naive, perhaps the nationwide eagerness to tell everyone the public national norms for sexual performance creates even further inadequacy and more need for the couch.

We seem to be a splendid breed for carrying on public display, whether we are reporting on the latest UFO, tying yellow ribbons around trees, or ourselves around a nuclear plant; or getting a hostile letter off to the local newspaper; or confiding on a national TV talk show what our great uncle did in the hayloft; or calling the local radio and abusing some issue. We hover on being a society where all the inmates are outside the asylum.

I know that many of my remarks only reflect the natural withdrawal and conservatism of becoming older, and I should be careful or I will get "hung up on my internalized tension." My thoughts and words are not bitter, not excessively aged. I make them because I think there is a silent majority, yes majority of us, who don't believe in group laundering any more than we believe in group sex. The columnists, the talk shows, the books, the movies -- all are exploiting the inadequacies and catering to the need by a few to be seen and heard. The essential core of the country does not see UFOs, does not abuse children, does not get reincarnated, does not hear voices or regularly converse with the departed.

The majority who go on about life's living and doing normal things in a normal way are submerged under the blitz and blather of all the media. We are an endangered species not because we are a minority, but because media dominate our external perception of ourselves. We aren't what we are, we hover on becoming what they say we are. A strange and dangerous circumstance.

58. Obits to Match Our Mountains

Comedian George Burns, still funny at near age 100, has a one-liner: "First thing I do when I get up in the morning is read the obituary column. If my name isn't in it, I have breakfast."

The audience enjoys this humor touched with irony as Mr. Burns takes a draw on his cigar, savoring it with their laughter.

Such lightheartedness is the expected easygoing style for handling the subject. Variations, all pure American, include: "Boy! What a hangover. I wish I was dead. In fact, I thought I was dead until I shaved. The bleeding reassured me."

We Americans seek this casual dealing with reality and can find cheerful variations from poets as well as comedians:

> Around, around the sun we go:
> The moon goes 'round the earth.
> We do not die of death:
> We die of vertigo.
>
> --Archibald MacLeish
> *"Mother Goose's Garland"*

All of which is an introduction to my main topic: the quality of obituaries and, especially, the dullness of medical obituaries.

Not only do American medical journals neglect the art of "summing up the career," but even when a journal does attempt an obituary, it is laundered, yawn-provoking, and gives no clue to the strengths and flaws, the moods and memories that were the woman or man.

I know readers will shake their heads and gently fume over this morbid concern with the obituary, but a life well-lived needs, deserves, some words of summary.

Some, of course, tell their own story, but not all of us get around to writing the autobiography -- an effort that could be defined as a reconstruction of what you did, obscuring what you did not -- or telling enough of the truth in the hope that history will overlook the truths not told.

We Americans enjoy our wit and humor about death, and yet, when the curtain is lowered, we get one inch in the newspaper with a list of offspring, and a closing line urging the reader to send money to the Heart Association.

The thought is morbid, but young, beginning physicians would do themselves a favor if they frequently read the obituaries in the English journals: *The Lancet* and the *British Medical Journal.*

The English do a first-class job of memorializing the lately departed. And, of course, all those on the waiting list, (living is 100 percent fatal) have satisfaction in knowing several hundred words will be placed in the permanent archives of the world's medical libraries, narrating, almost always in quite superior English, the landmarks of one's career.

The fact that such a written record will occur must have a positive influence on performance. Surely one works harder, more scrupulously, when the grand finale holds promise of several hundred words placed before all who read English.

This must have some positive persuasion when compared to the quite frugal, sterile, 20-word *JAMA* farewell.

The Lancet of course has superb grist. Englishmen have distinct advantages: they are born in exotic-named places where the Empire seconded their father, they serve their Queen in far-off places; they are mentioned in dispatches.

Relish these samples: "When war was declared he joined the Royal Army Medical Corps and became advisor in medicine to the Malta Command throughout the siege and was awarded the OBE for his services there."

In peace, the vocabulary is equally elegant: " ... he was honorary physician to the Queen. He was an officer of the Venerable Order of St. John of Jerusalem."

The Lancet does not hesitate to give color to the departed: "He was a character. He had a strong and well-known fuse and abhorred the progressive erosion of moral standards in post-war years. His annoyance and frustration occasionally boiled over into rages."

Another example: "A great supporter of the weak or poor, his tenacity and conviction made him a difficult and sometimes infuriating colleague and reduced his effectiveness in committees. He could be short-tempered and severely critical of those who failed to meet his own high standards. He taught through criticism."

There! Those are real characters, warts and all. When some future person wants to know what old Dr. Cedric Figglebody was all about, *The Lancet* has it all spelled out.

Just this day *The Lancet* comes, and I quickly turn to my favorite section: "He was not a handsome sort, but was aristocratic in appearance and autocratic by nature; he was a better talker than listener."

Another: "He was a discriminating gourmet and a superb raconteur. ... In middle life he took up skiing and through sheer strength and foolishness became fast but not graceful ... because of his marvelous sense of fun and his strange recall of the ridiculous he could be guaranteed to enliven any after-dinner speech, even if he was not delivering it." I love that!

These are but samples of why it may be delightful to live in the United States -- but one should give serious consideration to dying in England. The obit may be worth it.

59. Verbal Speed and Obsolescence

Columnists Edwin Newman and William Safire write delightfully about the misuses, changes, abuses of the English language as it is Americanized.

The growth of the American-English vocabulary through the invention of new words make archaic an education acquired in the 1920s. How could one communicate, even exist, if one did not have the essential vocabulary? "T.V., credit card, satellite, floppy disk, hot tub, four-on-the-floor, ballpoint, jet, hi-fi, blow-dry, microwave, hugger jeans, shades, give me five, on-line?" Was there communication prior to this?

None of this concerns me. I enjoy the energy of our American version of English. New words, new ideas, new expressions are a dividend of a vigorous society. Changes in grammar and usage don't pain me as they do Mr. Newman and Mr. Safire. English was never a fixed science; each era leaves behind its bit of language residue.

No, none of this worries me. What does catch my attention is not these small written language issues. I am concerned only when I find that the actual spoken language called English has been transformed as it is used in daily verbal communication.

This first came to my attention through frequent contacts with my then 26-year-old daughter. My telephone would ring, and although I would recognize the voice, I had no idea what she said. It was a matter of velocity. This daughter, raised in an era of TV commercials, has a record rate of verbal velocity.

Commercials cost vast sums. Fifteen seconds of

TV advertising time is frequently all a major company buys. To make maximum their 15 seconds, not only are the words spilled out without inhaling, but 15 colorful scenes zip across the screen and a pack of musicians pound in the background. The product's name flashes on and off. The spoken voice is only a part of the imprinting tactic.

When my daughter spoke to me on the phone, her mind was racing against the 15-second cut-off. Her experiences with TV had left her with the expectation that I was not only hearing her machine-gun delivered message, but undoubtedly I was hearing music, seeing slides, and her kernel message was flickering before my eyes.

I developed a protective approach. When the 15-second barrage ended, I quite politely said, "What did you say?" I did not confuse the issue by saying we had a bad connection or my hearing was failing, or counterattack with "Speak English!" Simply, "What did you say?" This was an acceptable question because commercials are supposed to be repeated, identically, rapidly, frequently. My daughter, letter-perfect, made the same sounds, repeating them two or three times.

We never quarreled or exchanged hostile criticisms, but it was obvious to both of us that the distance between our generations was in part a matter that I spoke American-English, and she spoke 15-second phonetic tele-English. Our generation gap was not the 40 years separating us, it was that she was able to say hundreds of words in 15 seconds, which certainly is impressive.

Then I took a granddaughter on a cruise ship. A 50-year generation gap. We were together every day. Each other's only company. In other words, we had to communicate with each other. I had a superb chance to analyze further this new means of communication.

My granddaughter has moved on beyond my daughter. She is the full flower of this new phonetic medium. There is no punctuation, no sentence ends, no word is discreet and, in this new, more complete version, no inflection.

I watched my granddaughter's face, lips, facial movements. The lips were slightly apart, but nothing else moved. Lip-reading was useless, impossible. All phonation was inside, resolved between tongue and sinuses. She said to me one morning, Wateyagonadutay."

This was said to me, I know, because no one was near us, and it had to be me to whom she was speaking. Her head was turned, eyes elsewhere. The voice was absolutely flat, no rising or falling. Not a flicker of movement to the lips. Total time for this communication was slightly under one second. With my silence, she repeated: "Wateyagonadutay," this time looking at me for reinforcement.

With a flush, the meaning came to me. I was able to stop thinking of American-English and instead, I swept my mental computer bank for these sounds. Just as one can hear a few musical notes and from some tucked away brain-store, exclaim, "Why, that's *Old Man River!*" I mastered this monotone, exhaled, apunctuated, non-inflected query: "What are you going to do today!" The rest of the cruise was a joy. I stopped listening for content. I sought only the sound, and then ran it through my head until I had a match. "Duahavtaetit." This was always said with the appetizer at dinner: "Do I have to eat it?" Granddaughter had been raised on fast food. She had never seen capers and cold salmon.

"Ilebeelatrthnlasnite." This was always said as she went off to the late-evening dancing: "I'll be later than last night." My ears now receive at this rate, but I don't speak this way, my lips can't handle it.

The uninitiated may claim that this is a teen-age variant, and with time it passes. Does age and duty slow this verbal velocity? Years after this cruise, with her college degree done, and a husband in hand, I sent her a gift. The phone rang and without any preamble I heard: "Grndadythanxfrthmony." Ah! sweet music.

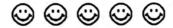

60. On Hard Work and On Being 'Educated'

I was browsing through papers and came across an article by Mortimer Adler, the guru of Great Books, who took on the subject of "updating" his list of Great Books. He identifies the roster of printed, blue-ribbon source material that he and Robert Hutchins published in 1952, the Great Books, that has served as a guide for self-education for more than 25 years. Now, as this century moves to its end, Adler suggests it might be possible to update the 1952 list with something of merit from this century. In this article regarding great books, Adler updates his original list, which stopped with 1899, and weighs authorship of our century.

Adler seems almost resistant to the thought that something worthwhile may have been written in the 20th century. After verbal hesitations and disclaimers, he compromises by dividing the 20th century into two parts: 1900 to the end of World War II -- which he feels may have enough aging to make value judgments valid -- and the second period from 1945 to the present -- which he thinks is still too soon to give a critic's honest perspective.

I won't try to recite all the works that Adler places his imprimatur on, although it is a provocative list, but here are the authors of what he considers the lasting creative literature of the first 45 years of this century: first, of course, George Bernard Shaw, then James Joyce, Marcel Proust, Thomas Mann, D. H. Lawrence, William Faulkner, T. S. Eliot, Franz Kafka.

When I saw those names, I knew I was in trouble. In fact, I was falling rapidly from the ranks of literate men. For I knew his selection was heavily weighted with much of the very literature I have constitutionally been unable to enjoy.

I reached my educable manhood in these very years upon which Adler gives judgment, and I failed the course. No matter how I tried, nor how substantial the critics' accolades, I have some biochemical fault, perhaps a missing enzyme, and I could not when young, nor again when middle-aged, nor now, a seasoned wanderer on the high plateau, enjoy, savor, enthuse over, nor persuade myself that I cared for James Joyce, Marcel Proust, D. H. Lawrence, or Franz Kafka.

More than six times I have pulled *Ulysses* from the shelf and beat my way through its staccato flashes (and, to me, psychopathological passages) and could only feel a concern for the stability of the author. In fact, it was that circumstance, the probable pathology of the author, which made it even possible for me to have any knowledge about these authors. Many of them have a high level of odd, eccentric, aberrational behavior, and I have enjoyed, as a physician, learning something of their life stories. Yes, the authors' own careers make good reading because of their excessive behavior, but their writings I don't need.

Just to be sure I have not unknowingly acquired more depth and have now reached the necessary level of perception not achieved before, I re-read the first four chapters of *Ulysses*. I voiced no opinion, but persuaded my wife, a scholarly woman, to do the same. She read the first chapter and announced with some pride, "I think I understand some of it. There evidently are three men up in a tower, but I don't know why they are there, and what they are trying to say, or what their relationships are, one to each other." She did not volunteer to read further, but I can vouch for the inexplicable message of the next three chapters. *Ulysses* went back on the shelf, still too sick for this doctor's attention.

I felt less lonely, immersed in my illiteracy, when an article appeared in the *British Medical Journal*, in its column titled, "Reading for Pleasure." This essay, contributed by an English physician, was identified as "A Journey with Proust." I believe I have found a kindred illiterate, or a kindred honest man. He says of Proust: " ... his work is safely in the category of classic defined as books everyone would like to have read, but no one wants to read." A good definition of some of the material on Adler's list.

Among my friends there are physicians, many of them are very successful -- successful in how effectively to serve mankind -- and many of them are as unappreciative of these authors as I. The "reading" desires of my physician colleagues, by and large (and that is too broad a statement, I know) simply do not allow them to savor this list blessed by Mortimer Adler. *Ulysses, The Cocktail Party, The Wasteland, Sons and Lovers, The Trial, Remembrance of Things Past*, are all of the genre of heavy-handed psychological viewings of mankind -- and, if not of mankind, of the author. A viewing that most physicians don't need. The reality of the situation is that such writings, if they are what a civilized man or woman should read, leave a very large number of intelligent, contributing, useful citizens uneducated.

I know I am speaking far too broadly, and there are of course skilled, committed physicians who have had great joy from *Ulysses* -- and I acknowledge I don't know at all well the reading range of women physicians -- I am comfortable with the point I am making: a definition of a civilized, educated physician that makes it necessary that one has immersed ones self in credit courses in Proust, T. S. Eliot, D. H. Lawrence, Franz Kafka, for example, will make most of us fail the definition. One suspects that beyond the closed coterie of critics, that many might fail this test.

I do not include George Bernard Shaw, for I can read his creations with satisfaction. I hesitate to include William Faulkner, who is also on Adler's list -- because I can enjoy a modest dose of Faulkner and appreciate some of his intense characterizations -- but a small dose is all. I simply have no need for all of the unhappy psychopaths that he manages to weave into the dark, shadowed reaches of Mississippi. As I have said, I do enjoy the biographies of these authors, for they certainly lived, most of them, intemperate, interesting lives. Thomas Mann is almost beyond belief, for he evidently was a normal, logical person.

Lord Russell Brain, in writing the forward to Cooper's *The Quiet Art: A Doctor's Anthology,* said: "The doctor occupies a seat in the front row of the stalls of the human drama, and is constantly watching, even intervening in, the tragedies, comedies, tragicomedies that form the raw material of the literary art." That says exactly what I want to convey; I am sorry I didn't say it first. A physician lives these experiences in real life. There is little space left, little emotional capacity left, for the meanderings of the author who works out in a novel his own problems.

Is my feeling regarding these authors based simply on the fact that they are too close to my own time and experience? Do I do better as a civilized, educated physician if I go back to the original Great Books of Adler and Hutchins, the gleanings of 2,500 years? Maybe yes, maybe no. Leaping out from that list are three books I have just now gone to my shelves, yes, I own them, and pulled down to riffle through. These are truly the Great Books, for they are on the list of all great literature -- literature cited as that which must be read by anyone who claims a status as "broadly" educated.

The three books I have beside me are first,

Milton's *Paradise Lost*, second, Dante's *Inferno*, and third, Bunyan's *Pilgrim's Progress*. I looked through them, tried again to read them, as I have so many times -- and again put them down. No, I again failed. I ask myself, "Is this evidence that I lack a certain sensitive perception of greatness? Do I lack the intellectual apparatus to understand these three always-cited foundations of civilized reading? Or am I finally old enough, secure enough in my own ability to understand, that I can close these three books and happily, blithely say that I have not the slightest interest in them, never have, and never will? I am highly suspicious that many who put them on their list of obligated reading if one is to be called "educated", probably never read them either. Give yourself a test -- pick up *Paradise Lost* -- and tonight, after dinner, in a comfortable chair and in comfortable clothes, begin at the beginning -- and read it through. Before you do, make arrangements with someone to awaken you. *Paradise Lost* is written Halcion. I am of course confident Milton read it -- but it enters my mind that not many have read it who are alive today -- and if they did read it, they did so because it was required in a course. Anyone who claims his knowledge, sensitivity, understanding, or that anything was enhanced because of it, is on my suspect list.

With most of it behind me, I wonder if a great deal of what is defined as the necessities of an educated mind is not considerably in need of winnowing. Winnowing out is made difficult because the academic world's determination to analyze the psyche of Joyce, Lawrence, and Kafka distracts rational thought almost as much as Freud disturbed our ability to be different but normal, and stay free of his labels.

I drift peripheral to my point: Six or eight years of a young life, well-used, prepares one to be a safe and civilized physician. *Prepares only*, for the education is a continuing, unremitting experience which lasts for the lifetime. A lifetime in which one judges what completes his or her education. Long enough to admit that Dante's *Inferno* has never been part of that plan.

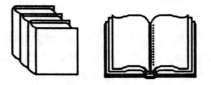

61. Care and Maintenance of the Body

A familiar term, a way of identification, is for medical school faculty members to refer to the entire group of students as "The Student Body". That is a convenient means of lumping off all students as if all the individuals were a single entity, instead of a complicated mix of age, race, background, gender, religion, and intelligence. The only homogeneity, the only common denominator, is that this "Body" intends to become a physician to the national "Body", the people. That is a unifying, tie that binds relationship, and this essay is written in that spirit.

Is there any message one could send from here on the Hill that could relate to the well-being of all who make up the "Student Body"? One could ask, playing cutely with modern language, is there a body language that could serve all? Are there aphorisms, gleanings, distillates that seem to me the truth? This does not mean that I knew they were the truth when I was their age. Living is an education. Life is a school house. I took all the courses. I think I have passed all the examinations given, some by repeating, and if not *cum laude*, am at least able to sit on a hill, reasonably serenely. Sit here happily, and with no obvious regrets. The regrets are well hidden.

Put this in your followup files, and in 2055, when you will be just about my age, look it up and see if you have learned the same lessons. Of course, by making the same mistakes.

1. You are born with a machine, a body, and whether you like it or not, it is one you are going to live with --

and die with.

2. This body cannot be traded in and it must be maintained if you are to be.

3. Your parents made this body. Be grateful they got you here. Be grateful for the launching they gave you. If you don't succeed in life, don't saddle your parents with criticism about how they are the problem. It is your life, your mind, your character, your personality. If you succeed, be generous with your compliments about your origins. If you fail, made foolish choices, and are inadequate, don't reach back and hang the fault on your mother and father.

4. Your body needs maintenance. The rules are simple. Stay skinny. All the fancy diets and clever books cannot improve on those two words. Stay fit. Not too fit. It may seem logical that you will be healthier if you run 20 miles a week, or more. Your body doesn't need that trauma. Your knees and hips don't need to be put through that. Working out on weights may give you pectorals but those are useless for the long haul. Leanness, mobility, agility are what you seek. Exercise may give you a way to burn off your tensions, your stress, your catecholamines -- but that can be golf, or tennis, or a wood shop. If you really want to take on a life time "sport", go for swimming. It meets all the requirements. Or walking. Pick something that can fit your way of life -- for a lifetime.

5. Don't be a fool and acquire a nicotine addiction. Don't tolerate yourself being stuck with something that absolutely is going to affect your health. If you are one already addicted, clean up your act. You have only one body to go the route. Don't confuse the facts

by claiming that smoking relaxes you, lifts you -- just admit you are an addict and you need to go through detoxification. Get it done. Now.

6. Live more frugally that you need to. Drive a lesser car than you need to. Count on living to at least 80 and from the earliest possible moment, as you begin having an income, plan to be old -- and with a happy financial base. You and The Body may be in great shape at 70, but you will be in better shape if you have spaced your finances to go the route.

7. Pay attention to finances. Be a thoughtful caring physician, be generous with your abilities, give your efforts to those who need you -- but protect your family. Protect your family so the children can have an education equal to yours, so you and your spouse can enjoy the whole span, but don't feel an obligation to create a financial dynasty. You are in the wrong profession if your goal is wealth.

8. Don't wreck your children by making it unnecessary for them to work as hard as you have. Give them love, an education that fits their talent, and get out of their way.

9. Consider the merits of marriage, but not too early. Life is long and there is much to do and learn. Some of the lessons can be learned best, enjoyably, single. Some are improved by marriage. Allot sufficient parts of your life to both experiences.

10. Keep discovering yourself. These years in getting through medical school and residency may seem to be a sufficient opportunity. Don't accept this as your limits. Remain a physician, think like a physician, but explore your potential. Grow. Make a right angle

turn once or twice in your career. Surprise yourself. Have some adventures. Live a bit dangerously, carefully.

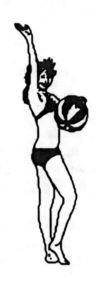

62. Some Secrets

It may be difficult to believe this, but one does learn certain things by living. Awareness, maturity, understanding are linear. They grow over a lifetime. Older people can offer valid thoughts about life; experience does have value. When young, few can believe this. Or one assumes that he or she is different and no other experience can match their problems. Perhaps that is true. I led my own life a little too much by this attitude. However, when one is at the other end of the run, it is permissible to have an opinion.

Things you will learn:

• You are not required to do what is popular. Don't devalue yourself because you do not enjoy joining a large, enthusiastic, happy mob such as the 70,000 at a football game, the crowd waiting at the terminal for the return of the team, the throngs lining a parade route, a yowling mob in a bar. Perfectly normal, well-adjusted people can find such mob-enthusiasm not their cup of tea. Don't consider yourself anti-social if you are at your best in a small one-on-one setting.

• You are not a misfit if you do not squeal, swoon and faint when seeing "famed" popular musicians. At the other end of the spectrum, one may well find grand opera boring. Many offerings by famous symphony orchestras produce somnolence. One can be perfectly normal and not enjoy any of these. One may be absolutely healthy and still not like to have the radio on, the television playing, or a headset applied to the ears. One may truly enjoy silence.

• Don't feel clod-like, clumsy, and essentially un-American if you do not do sports of any sort gracefully, if you do not know how to dance, and cannot activate your feet and body to the rhythm of music. Being able to be agile and dexterous is not a requirement for original and creative thought. Perfectly good, normal, happy people sit in chairs and do their best work, thinking, chatting, with one or two others, or even alone. Yes, including talking.

• Don't fault yourself if you do not enjoy joining a laughing, boisterous, gaily happy group of hugging, back-slapping, witty-remarks tossing enthusiasts. Conviviality can be one-on-one. It is not necessarily a group effort. Perfectly normal and happy people cannot like such gatherings and yet have a full range of emotions but present them quietly and privately.

• Don't consider yourself a wall-flower, a drab sparrow, if you do not have a great need for the latest in style, hair-cut, make-up, car, and gadgets. Large numbers of people find their own style of dress, their hair-style, and go through life quite happily. Driving a car that does not "express" yourself is not evidence you are not alive and well. Being stable, steady, the same, is not a bad way to be. Perfectly normal people look and dress the same when they are 30 as when they are 60. New gadgets are new gadgets. They should not be confused with functional trusted allies such as a razor, or umbrella, or belt, or old clothes, or stethoscope -- things that have been part of yourself for many good years.

• Don't fault yourself as unintelligent if you really cannot devote an evening to a card game. Bridge and poker are not an index by which to judge your real ability. People who play those games may have their character faults, too, and you must not allow them to shadow your character by their smugness. The same is true with golf. Golf playing is not evidence of a superb character. It is not necessary to be able to play golf, or bridge, or poker, or Scrabble, or Monopoly, or tennis, nor be a dancer, to be a very useful, valuable citizen. Remember that.

• Don't feel hollow and empty if you do not know how to cook, how to barbecue; or enjoy hanging on every word in the menu, salivating over the description of each sauce. Do not feel second-level, rural, if you really do prefer a glass of the house wine to some inordinately priced French wine that has sediment in the bottle. Perfectly normal people can enjoy plain food, digest it, keep their weight down, keep barbecue spots off their shirt, and still succeed in this world. One can live an entire life, live it well, live it exuberantly, in fact, and know very little about cordon bleu food and the right wine.

• Don't consider yourself expendable if you really do not like weddings, church services, testimonials, service clubs, pledges to the flag, barber shops, dirty jokes, profanity. Perfectly normal, useful citizens, valuable citizens, may never be in a church, may never picket, may never use a dirty word, may be bored by the people who do all these things, and still be socially graceful, kind, caring, and not an embarrassment to their family.

• Don't feel inadequate because you cannot do any of the above, do not want to do the above, and when doing the above are restless and anxious to get back to real life. Perfectly normal happy people can be quiet, modest, and enjoy solitude. They can even be good parents. The country is not harmed by them.

But, you had better be energetic, dedicated, directed, caring, and have perseverance beyond all else. These are the qualities that begin to single out the achievers, the contributors, the leaders. All the above are just variations on window dressing, a part of the background -- but not the reason you are here.

63. Age 70

That noise I hear is my somatic clock, tocking away evenly -- but away. December 8, 1918 was a time of high excitement, for World War I had ended not a month earlier, and all lives were readjusting. My arrival undoubtedly produced a little readjustment and perhaps a little excitement, at least for my mother, for I arrived on her birthday. Whatever enthusiasm my parents felt, it was enough to conclude their parenting. I remained an only child.

By 70, one may acquire a degree of wisdom. If I had known I would reach age 70, I would have paid more attention to wisdom along the way.

There's a fine line between wisdom and carping. All wisdom is not shining, some hurts.

One doesn't get wisdom without mistakes, but a lifetime of mistakes makes one wrong, not wise. Corrected mistakes become wisdom.

Wisdom is not a male possession: old men enjoy acting wise; senior women are wise.

One may have a fortune and a large reputation and still be a fool. Wisdom and high position are not always paired. Some of the wisest people one meets are those who are not willing to trade away their convictions for popularity.

Successful people are not necessarily the wisest people.

Fame and respect are not the same thing. Be suspicious of fame.

Life is fleeting, but there is no alternative. The years you have are your only real possession, invest well. Be jealous of them. Listen, observe, query, but be cautious of another's advice; no one else knows all the variables you are weighing. Counsel yourself.

Be the same today as yesterday. Don't cause those around you to wonder what mood you will have today; you owe those around you a pleasant face. The facade is what the world sees, the private you hums along inside, steady, on course, weathering storms, making judgments, learning, handling stress. Maturity is stress management.

Study history. Travel wisely. Understand how tribes, religion, economy, ambition have flowed across the earth's geography. Read the daily news, but read in-depth separately and teach yourself the layers of history behind current events. Be suspect of public announcements, and ask yourself what are the unstated influences behind the events. If you're being manipulated, at least know it.

Ignore the message that you mustn't work too hard. If you choose the right career, working hard is what you will want to do. You have a very few decades of very high energy, dependable health and opportunity; use them by using them entirely. There is plenty of time yet for coasting, but the prime years are for doing, and doing means building reputation, building family, learning who you are.

Get up early, work hard all day, go to bed tired. Don't pollute yourself. Before you are 70, you will have a collection of old acquaintances who fell by the wayside because of alcohol. Why wait until 70 to learn that? Believe in living right. Lean, keen, smokeless decades will not deprive you of good living; instead, you will gain good living, out beyond 70.

Have long-range plans. Anything worth doing will require at least 10 years to do well. Avoid short-range tasks. When a project is done, a plan accomplished, know when to break. Master making right-angle turns. You won't know what your range of ability is unless you explore what's around the corner. Don't stay too long on any stage; make clean breaks which don't need excuses. Turn from what you were doing on your own time schedule, not by the push of others.

A few friends are enough. The very few from childhood will last surprisingly well. Add a few during your active years, and the best of these friends may be completely unrelated to your profession. Plan it so your children become your best friends and they join the special circle along with your childhood friends.

Among the friends, put a few pets. A dog, cat, horse, properly cultivated and respected, can occupy vast areas of your inner aloneness.

Don't take yourself too seriously, but don't be trivial. Laugh easily, but laugh even more when you're alone. When you find they are laughing at you, stop, take stock -- you are treading on quicksand.

Live and enjoy the day, but remember, ages 40, 50, 70 are coming; enjoy this day, but the other days will come sooner than you think. Lay aside resources for these later years -- resources of reputation and money, but also the gleanings of thoughtful reading and broad study.

Be honest. You'll have enough problems in life just from living. Don't compound them by chicanery, cheating, lying.

One has to be careful with wisdom. Its greatest merit is when it is kept inside and is used to guide your own conduct. Wisdom becomes suspect when one offers it as I am doing here.

Don't overestimate your experience and knowledge. You are alive and learning until it ends. You are still unfinished.

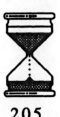

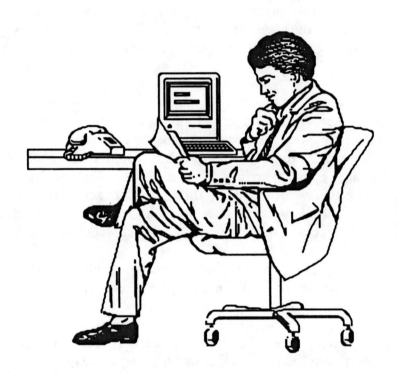

Printed in the United States
102669LV00004B/351/A